Peace Therapy
"The Healing Process Begins"

2nd Book of Storoems
by
Renzie

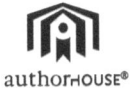

authorHOUSE®

AuthorHouse™
1663 Liberty Drive, Suite 200
Bloomington, IN 47403
www.authorhouse.com
Phone: 1-800-839-8640

First published by AuthorHouse 1/30/2009

ISBN: 978-1-4389-0111-4 (sc)
ISBN: 978-1-4389-0112-1 (hc)

Printed in the United States of America
Bloomington, Indiana

This book is printed on acid-free paper.

Table of Contents

My Apology

Before any pages are turned, any words are read, I offer you *(the reader)* my deepest apology for not giving you a better quality of work in my previous book. By doing that, I did not give you the best of my gift and for that I sincerely apologize. Like so many others I tried walking before crawling, thinking I could do it on my own, and not using the help that was there waiting for my call, the one that never came. My promise now is to give you the type of writing that will heal, help, guide and dazzle your mind, body and soul; and if nothing else, help you grow spiritually and mentally.

"Renzie"

Dedication

Once again I've been asked to dedicate my work.

Whoever came up with the idea of dedication has made it hard on writers, especially when there are so many candidates, but this one was easy.

I dedicated this book to GOD (my Heavenly Father and my mother (my Earthly Angel).

To my Heavenly Father, there really is no need to go into detail because you know how grateful and thankful I am for what you have blessed me with and will bless me with, from the cell to the egg and no doubt, your mercy and grace. Words can not say what you mean to me, so I ask you to look at my heart. To my Earthly Angel, people want to know where it all comes from; they need to look no further than you and your life, the perfect example in my eyes. The amount of love I have for you can not be measured. So, from me to the both of you, I say this, our bond will never be broken and my love for you continues to grow. I love you both, from the day of the thought, to the day of rest.

Acknowledgements

As you know this portion of the book is to acknowledge those who have made it possible for the book being written. Those who have inspired me, those who have pushed me when I felt I couldn't go on, those who have carried me when it seemed my burden was too much for me to bare. I acknowledge those who didn't give up on me, those who prayed for me and had those prayers answered. I acknowledge those who cried with me as I cleaned out my closet, because part of them was in there and they couldn't move on until I moved out and on. And most of all, those I love. So only one name will be mentioned, all others will fall in the category of Family, Friends or Enemies.

So without further ado, I acknowledge my Lord and Savior, Jesus Christ, because without him none of this would be possible. And for those who will remain nameless, know that you have given me what was and is needed to write any book or in my case, to tell our stories. So when you read a sentence or phrase and think that it's about you, then it probably is about you, so I thank you in advance.

It's time for us to move on and when I take a step forward, I hope you take one, because it takes two steps to complete a walk, and that's what we'll be doing is walking together as one. I just hope that we're walking in the same direction. **Enjoy!!!!**

Introduction

I would like to start my introduction out by saying welcome to those who are reading my work for the first time, and to those who are continuing this journey with me, I say, "glad to see you again". While reading, you'll also be introduced to my style of writing known as **"Situation Writing"**.

As we enter into the second phase of discovering who we really are; what we want and how to get it. It's time to relax again; so kick off your shoes and grab a bottle of your favorite beverage. Let your hair down and free your mind. In order to travel to some of the places we're about to venture, you don't need to create anymore obstacles than you already have.

It has taken me forty years to reach the point where I am today. I'm finally learning how to express myself and the joy that comes with it. Not just joy for myself, but joy for others as well. It's my goal to brighten up someone else's day, to give guidance to someone who seems to have lost their way and just to be a shoulder for someone to lean or to cry on. This is truly a Blessing.

I have many to thank, so I won't mention any names, just know that I thank-you all, whether our experience was good or bad, it has helped me grow. I give praise and honor to GOD, who deserves all the credit, because I'm still here enjoying life and being blessed, all because of him.

It's time to heal!

Our Neighbors

We meet at the same place, same time, with the exception of those nights when they can't come out and play. We tell our stories to each other, as if we're talking to one of our sisters or brothers.

We're such wonderful friends; we listen to any and everything each other has to say. We pick each other up when we're down, without ever making a sound.

We sometimes see one of our neighbors taking a fall, but that's alright because they're answering a call.

Someone out there is in need of a friend; a prayer needs to be answered; a life needs to be brightening up. That's what true friends do, would you like to be one too?

So we'll say goodbye to one of our neighbors for the last time, as he's summoned to duty to bring light to the end of someone's tunnel, who's been in the dark long enough.

Does that mean neighbors are blessing? Yes it does, not all blessings are seen and miracles are not always understood or explained.

So tonight when we sit down and talk, I'll let them know you would like to join in. I'm sure they won't mine a new neighbor, from time to time.

Broken Spirit

It's known as "The Forbidden Place", so I don't suggest you vacation there, it's also a place you wouldn't want to take the family, not if you really care.

Native Americans say it's a horse you can't ride, and the peace pipe won't help you either, if you're looking for a place to hide.

We all have to deal with it at some point in time, and you're no different from the rest of us, so be quiet and just wait in line.

Others will notice the change, but won't say a word; they'll turn their heads and pretend to be looking at the birds.

But birds don't fly in office rooms, unless you've flown up the cuckoo's nest to make a deposit, because you think you'll be there soon.

That's just one indication of the screws being loose, another is walking around moping, hoping and joking that everything is alright, while deep within you, you know you're a sad sight.

What do you do? You won't tell anyone because you think they won't understand and think you're less than a man or woman.

That's when weakness is camouflaged by what you think is pride, but it's slowly breaking you down, stride by stride.

Eventually you'll let go, and that's when your one true friend will step in, and maybe, just maybe you'll realize he's always there, from the beginning to the end.

The Waiting Room

No one knows how long you'll be there, nor do they care.
If that was the case then we wouldn't be having this
conversation and the doctor wouldn't be prescribing you
medication.

So it seems you're just like the rest of us; dazed and confused
and don't know who to trust. That's why you were sent here,
to "The Waiting Room", it's time to clean house, but you
forgot your broom.

You've allowed your dirt, cob-webs and dust to accumulate
to such a degree they have no where else to go, except to live
among us.

We sit here waiting for someone to come to the window as
if their seeing a new addition to the family for the first time,
only to be reminded we've committed a crime; a crime of
passion, of unforgiving, of having a big ego, and a crime of
misunderstanding.

So we won't be going home with any families anytime soon,
and we're lucky our crime hasn't sent us to our doom. Now
you know someone out there still cares, because the end
hasn't come yet, only the cold hard stares.

Whispering Winds

Oh, how soothing they are, just close your eyes and let them take you for a ride. Silent at times, but that's just to let you soak up the moment.
Watching them blow the tall grass in the fields reminds me of waves crossing an ocean. I listen to them as they squeeze through the unseen cracks I know are there, but where?

Sometimes howling to get my attention, as if to ask, "Don't you hear me or do I need to intensify and blow a few things over to let you know I am to be admired and respected?"

With the whispering comes the sounds of freedom and a message they bring with them just for me. As I watch them walk through the forest bending trees and branches, I see peace in the falling leaves as they sail to the ground without making a sound.

I welcome their melodies of peace that relaxes me and at the same time makes my body shiver. As they blow the hair on my body, I wonder if there is anyone out there that enjoys their company as much as I do.

When their visit is over and everything has come to a standstill, I'll tuck the experience away until it's needed another day or I'm entrusted with their presence, but for now I'll watch their departure in amazement just as I watched their arrival.

If I Never Make It Home

If I never make it home, there's something I want you to
know.
You are, have been and will always be a part of me.
Wherever I am, you are, in my mind, body and soul.
You'll always be with me, even when this old body gets cold.

If I never make it home, there's something I want you to
know.
I have never loved anyone as much as I love you. This much
is true.
You have all of me, right down to the last drop of sweat.
My last breath is yours for the taking, just ask and you shall
receive.

You've given me enough joy to last a lifetime,
So no more tears whenever I leave.
Now is the time to smile and laugh, and think of all the
wonderful memories
We've shared together.

If I never make it home, there's something I want you to
know.
We have been blessed with two sons, a gift from above.
They're a part of me, just look and you will see.
It's my time to cry, so hold your head high and be proud, like
I know you are.

No matter what I accomplish in life, it will never add up to
you.
You're one of God's treasures; I was just lucky I found you.

Tell the boys, I did my best, to be the best Dad I could be, and there's
No need to worry because GOD has given them an angel for a mother.
So if I never make it home, there's no need to weep,
Because love is still here, even when I sleep.

Much is given; much is receive; so along the way;
remember to get on your knees.

The White Highway

My mind floats with the clouds as the wind blows and we travel along the white highway. What a beautiful sight to see as I gaze out of my window.

A sense of peace and relaxation comes over me, because one day, I know I'll have to travel that highway myself.

Angel's line up one behind the other, with their wings expanded as they float in mid air waiting for their number to be called.

Saint Peter's at the entrance standing proud and strong, to make sure things run smooth and nothing goes wrong.

The White highway stretches for miles and miles, with no end in sight, but the angels don't complain, they just keep heading towards the light.

Besides, there's no need to rush because time stands still for those who lived according to his will.

Soothing music fills the air, as Gabriel plays the harp, to let me know I'm almost there.
I'm so amazed at the faces I see; Moses, Abraham, Isaac, and look grand mommy's there too.

All dressed in white, laughing, joking and standing around with smiles on their faces and nothing to do. I guess that's what happens when paradise calls you.

Billboards along the white highway light up the sky like the morning sun; they too let me know I'm moments away from all the fun.

Traveling the white highway makes me happy and I can't wait until I get my chance to stand with St. Pete, at that golden gate!

The Eyes Have It

No need to say a word, your eyes tell it all; you're tired and
all alone and just need a shoulder to cry on.

They let me know when you're in need; of help,
encouragement, inspiration and maybe a little mediation.

They let me know when you need a hand to hold, when
you've been left out in the cold.

They tell me when you need a walk; to listen while someone
else talks; when you're in pain and on the verge of going
insane.

They're the windows of our soul that need to be clean as we
get old.
They let me know when you're happy and it's time to rejoice;
when you're hurting after making a bad choice.

They let me know when you're on cloud nine and
everything's fine.
They can be stained and broken as well, when your life is a
struggle and you're catching hell.

They sparkle when you're proud of the effort the kids made.
Some have been known to have fire in them, when there's
burning inside; to extinguish, the storm has to subside.

They come with automatic wipers that flush out the pain and
sorrow, so you can have your new tomorrow.

When the lights are no longer on, and you're in the dark,
they let you see by hearing and touching.

Some say you've been blessed because you don't have to see the evil or its birth, that lurks on this planet we call earth.

So as your eyes tell your life story, don't forget to give Him his glory.

Trying to Hide

No longer able to hide the pain that has taken control of my life. It has become a daily struggle to place one foot in front of the other because I know each step gets me closer to my destruction.

My blooming has stopped, so has my life as I know it. My shadow now walks beside me because it has seen my future and wants no part of it.

My will to continue is no longer a pleasure that greets me at every obstacle. I've let my insecurity reach an all time low, which makes me sometimes want to call it quits, but I can't give up, too many depend on me to be their foundation.

What can I do? What can I say? When they see I'm lost and don't know the way; to happiness, to forgiveness and all that other mess, I use to call my friend.

In this weakened state, I must find, I have to find the strength that's deep within this battered temple of mine. I can't give in because now my life really begins.

No more wandering in the wilderness without direction or protection. Cover me Lord for I'm too weak to do it myself. Wash me with your liquid sunshine, cleanse my body of the old interior and allow my soul to breathe again.

I'm tired and I can't carry this burden anymore, so I submit myself to you, hoping you restore, rebuild and heal this fragile structure I call a body.

Unable to act as if no one sees the pain I wear day to day; that obliviously has blocked my way and hinders my growth, my existence and my divine right to live according to the book of life.

Some way, some how, I must filter the poisonous elements that have polluted my body and now dictates my every move.

If I'm ever to have my name put back in His book, then I must change my lifestyle and pray He take a second look.

While I Was Waiting

While I was waiting a lot of things wandered through my head.
I'm leaving a war zone, and a lot of soldiers are dead.
They paid the ultimate prize for people like you and me to be free.
But when I get back home there'll still be demonstrations in the streets.

Not everyone understands why we had to go and why so many have to die. Was this war justified or was it another lie?
So the explaining has to be done, not to us, the soldiers, because we know why we're here, but to the families, who have lost love ones this past year.

Now I see my family as I walk off the plane, but they're crying,
and they don't look the same. It's me, I call out, and I'm here to stay.
But not knowing it's me they simply turn away.

I thought they would be happy to see me, on this glorious day.
But to my amazement something has gotten in their way.
As I look to the rear of the plane, I understood why they were afraid to look. They see coffins being unloaded, and this time it's not in a newspaper or book.

So while I was waiting, reality set in. It made me realize this too could be the end. As I awaken from my deep sleep and the tears and shaking stopped, I realize it was only a dream and there's no longer a need to scream.

I know tomorrow is not promised, so I'll enjoy life's treasure's as they are given. I'll cherish, adore and be thankful for them all, and I'll do all of this, "While I'm Waiting" for that call.

Beautiful

Forget about what Webster and his friends tell you it is, because man wrote those and believe me when I say it's not man made.

It's in the eyes of the believer; it's what they see and how they see it. Some believe its skin deep and it covers you from your head to your feet.

Sunrises, Sunsets, Rainbows and Waterfalls, Yes, beautiful is in them all. Pouring rain on the desert sands, melting snow in my hand, and yet, some people still don't understand. Still I must reiterate it has nothing to do with man.

Tropical Islands where steps have never been taken, Rain forests and the awaking of undiscovered creatures are beautiful, and it still has many more features.

The way a mother loves her children, the sacrifice of a man, just to see his child's smile, seldom seen but often performed.

Watching you, watching me, watching the many examples of beautiful that set's my mind free.

Seeing a mother struggle with a smile on her face, teaches me there are some things you have to do whether you want to or not, it also tells me most mothers have seen the outcome and that's the reason for the smile.

Butterflies dancing in the fields, bears serenading after a fresh kill, beautiful gives different types of thrills.

It's talking to my father and hearing him talk back to me. I ask you what could be more beautiful than that. Beautiful is what I choose to be and the legacy I would like others to see.

Beautiful, if you have any more magic left, is it alright if I keep it for myself?

"An empty wagon makes a lot of noise".

You're Family Too

It's often said that a friend in need, is a friend in deed, and you've proven that to be true time and time again.

As I open up to you and allow you to enter into my silent world and explore what seems to me, to be the weight of the world on my shoulders, you let me know that family doesn't necessarily have to come from mom and dad.

You tell me what I need to hear and not what I want to hear, as most entourages do. You never sugar coat the truth, when you help me wash away some of the stains I've accumulated over the years.

You help me hold my head up high, when I'm down in the dumps and on the verge of a cry. You've brightened up some of my darkest days when I couldn't see, and that's another reasons why you're so special to me.

You're my friend, my strong sista, who I lean on when times get rough. I love you because you're sweet and beautiful inside and out, and that will never be questioned, so have no doubt.

As I seek your advice and wisdom, to become the best person I can possibly be, you say and do things as only a family member can.
So I offer you my hand as we take this journey of mine together.

Just know that you're in my heart, and the beat is as strong as ever, thanks to the love you've given without even knowing. I've always believed that angels come in many different forms, are you sure you're not one?

Whatever the case, it's fine with me, because you'll always be a branch, on my family tree.

Coming of Age

Proud is what I am, when I think about the things you've done and how you've grown into the man you are today. Responsibility, you showed that at a very young age. That chapter of your life is complete, and you did very well, so I can turn that page.

I remember holding you in my arms as an infant and I vowed I would always be there for you whenever you needed me. The changing of diapers, heating bottles of milk and dressing you, were talents I became good at, and I'm happy I learned them while taking care of you.

Some of my happiest memories are seeing you smile and enjoying life. You're grown now, but I still see the little boy whose hand I held whenever we went somewhere together. The same little boy I wanted people to know was my baby brother.

I read about your achievements in sports as I traveled around the world. I don't have many regrets in my life, but one is not seeing you play more, and being there to celebrate with you. But someone had to protect the world so you could have the choice to play.

You've blossomed into a beautiful butterfly, it may not be the manly thing to say, but it's the right thing to say. I hope the sun continues to shine and brighten your day, like you brighten mine, what else can I say other than "I Love You", and you will always be our Boo!

Uncle Sam is what the boys call you, not to join the army but because they love you just as much as I do, and I hear it in their voices. You've come of age better than I hoped you would. I guess we can thank GOD for putting a lot of mom in us.

So know this little brother, and never forget, my arms are open wide, just like Jesus has his, so if you ever need a hug, just close your eyes and think of us.

Dedicated to baby brother, Samuel "Ace" Thomas

Boiling Point

Over and over it plays in my head, so I better leave this place before someone winds up dead. Heartache and memory are now best friends and they won't let me sleep, until I bring it to an end.

Laughter and smiles have disappeared as well, but my mind was too cloudy for me to tell. This can't be happening, I told myself it never would, but I'm not in control anymore, that much is clearly understood.

Hatred has come into my life and it's very demanding. I know when it finishes, not even I'll be left standing. When you've went too far in whatever you did, it has a way of bringing you back home and making you fill like a kid.

No need to ask for help now, I missed all the signs as I traveled this road. Too late to put on the brakes, now it's time my story is told. Let's hope they don't make a movie, because I'll have to play the fool. Who else would they get to play the fool, who else but me?

I've visualized the scenes and it's not a pretty sight. My marriage, my life, is coming to an end, all because of the way I treated my best friend. When your best friend brings other family members into your fights, if that's what brought you to this point, simply know there's no future together and the end of your relationship is in sight.

I've reached the point where an explosion or eruption is about to take place. I must be prepared for what's about to begin. Hopefully I'll survive and one day, be able to call someone else my best friend.

The Closet

The Good Book tells us it's wherever you choose to go at that time when you've tried to figure it out on your own and it didn't work.

It's where you go when you acknowledge him, which you should have done in the first place, but you thought you had the key to open the door, because of the way you've been living your life.

It can be anywhere you choose it to be, all you have to do is close your eyes and give him a call, and he'll answer, because he doesn't consider any problem too small.

It's the one place you can really be yourself, you can cry and not worry about anyone seeing you, if that's what stopped you from going before.

Often we hang things up in there and forget about them. We sing without the use of a microphone and no one's there to judge us.

Storing things there because we think no one will find out what we did or it's too small and don't deserve your attention at the moment.

Some of them you can walk in and just pull out one problem at a time, others only have room enough for you to reach your arm in, because you've let your problems accumulate and now you really need help.

If I may, let me have the last say and give you a little advice. For most of us it's a place to fall on your knees and tell our deepest and darkest secrets. It's a place where we have that one-on-one conversation with our father without any interruptions.

It's been called a meeting or gathering place; a place you go to find the answers when you're confused and don't have a clue about what you should do. Most of us just call it our **"Closet"**.

It Finally Came Around

Too late to go back and change the hands of time, what's done is done, but it was ok when you were having your fun.

Now the shoe is on the other foot, you're at the end of your rope, what goes around has came, and when it's finished with you, you won't be the same.

They tried to tell you to stop before it was too late, but you didn't listen; now you have to eat what's on your plate.

Pack your bags, you're about to take a trip. I only hope it's a round trip ticket and not one way.

You made this mess and now it has flipped flopped. Now you say you found Jesus, but that's only because you want the pain to stop.

What's done in the dark soon comes to light, and that closet door you thought was closed, guess what? Peek-a-Boo, I see you!

Time to pay the piper and he doesn't take checks. You put a down payment way back when you thought your shit didn't stink.

It'll only happen once and it doesn't matter if you're a boy or girl, man or woman. It's not bias, never was, never will be. You don't have to take my word for it; you'll soon see.

You might as well get a handicap sign so everyone will know. No matter how hard you try to hide it, your life has just become a sideshow.

It's not the end of the world, but you may wish for it, after the aging process is over and the pain has subsided; just remember what you went through and how you got there; sometimes in order to get you right, your life has to give you a little scare.

Sometimes the sun shines at night.

Today I Saw an Angel

I saw an angel ascend today and I know Heaven was rejoicing. The angels were rolling out the golden carpet and preparing the angel walk. Earth is left with one less amazing person who's being rewarded for a job well done.

Afraid to die and wanting to cry; I'm expecting the worst, I won't lie. But I'll celebrate and won't put a damper on this occasion that's meant to be enjoyed.

I saw an angel today and it waved at me, as if to say don't worry, your day will come and I'll see you when you get here. A feeling of relief as well as grief, because I don't know when that day is coming, but I'll be happy when it does.

What a thing of beauty to see, an angel gliding in mid air as if it was riding an escalator in an upward direction. Yes, I saw an angel today and it made me smile for a while and forget my troubles.

Today's events no matter how strange they seem, gives me hope and allows me to dream that I too can be that angel someone will see ascending on a cloud. I saw an angel today and it saw me, and I realized that how I live my life is the key.

Falsifying Glory

There you go again trying to sell that lie. How long will you do it, I hope not until you die. A smile as big as the moon; a smile that will eventually, send you to your doom.

You prance around your friends at work, as if nothing is wrong and hope they don't notice your weakness, because they think you're strong.

Disguising your voice when talking to family members, being careful not to give them any clues, knowing later you'll crawl up in a corner and sing the blues.

Morning will come and the movie will start again, who will you play today, "The enemy within"? Praising GOD, when you know the devil is your best friend. If I were you I'd drop to my knees and try to make amends.

But you won't because your so-called pride wants you to stay, so you let your blessings slip away.

You don't have to live this lie anymore, just ask for help and he'll show you the door. It'll be tough without a doubt, but with GOD helping you, I think that's more than enough clout.

The Unauthorized Meeting

As he entered the room, silence filled the air, because he didn't know why he was there. I pretended to be writing and deep in thought, hoping he wouldn't be too mad, because it was his advice I sought.

Why did you request this meeting he asked, as if he didn't already know; because I have other places to go?

I shouldn't have to talk to you for another four to five years; do you think I'm supposed to come every time you're in tears?

You mean you really don't know why you're here; but you're "He who knows all", that has always been clear.

You're the one who sits on the throne, that I don't question. But this is one of those things I can't figure out on my own.

Enough chit-chat he said, get to the point and be brief, there's others who also need relief. I have countries to shake, cities to flood and thirsts to quench. Don't you watch the news, so don't call me every time you get the blues.

This is one time you'll have to find the answer yourself. I've given you what you need; it's in the black book that's covered in dust, just clean it off, read it and give me your trust.

Doubt will fade away, your troubles will leave, and all you have to do is simply believe.

Mourning Sickness

It's only supposed to last nine months, ten at the most; but it's
been two years and I'm still the host. I didn't know men went
through this as well, until the pain hit me and all I could do
is yell.
The anxiety comes and goes throughout the day, even my
family members try to stay out of my way.
Eating has become a difficult task, I crave for this, crave for
that, then I look in the mirror and it tells me I'm fat.
That's just another reason for me to tell someone off and
speak my mind, no one will say anything because their tired
of me mopping around and they just want things to be fine.

Everyone's nice to me because they think they know what
I'm going through, but they really don't have a clue
.

The kids go in the other room, when I come around. As if I'm
not already feeling bad.
Others in my life try to cheer me up, but they don't know the
real reason I'm in distress, they just think I need to rest.

Getting hungry in the middle of the night, but pickles and
ice cream won't do any good; I've even tried knotting on
wood.

Everyone thinks they know what I need, but this sickness
is not in books and not taught in schools, this is one of life's
lessons and you have to play by its rules.
I'm going to need more than just my friends, to heal these
wounds of mine and somehow make amends.

I've talked to doctors, Big Mommy and even the Pastors, I
think it's time I sought the real Master; he has always been
there for me, even when I was wrong.

He didn't have to, but I'm glad he was.

Maybe now, with his help, this mourning sickness will end and I can rejoice again with all my friends!

I Thought I Was Your Favorite?

You said if I do this, you would do that. Now you know, I would never, ever question your authority, but can you tell me what's going on?

I don't mean to sound arrogant or bossy, but you said if I followed your words, you would bless me.

I know you're not going back on your word, because it's written in stone. So can you please, pretty please, pick up the phone?

Uh oh, I hear thunder and see lightning on the horizon, but there isn't a cloud in sight, did I say something wrong, is that why you're uptight?

If I did, then I apologize, but this is someone who thirsts for your love, someone who feels weak when I'm not in your company.

This is someone who desires the peace only you can give; someone who loves you from the bottom of their heart, to the depths of their soul.

You give me the words I speak, so I couldn't have said the wrong thing. Maybe it's the way I said it, but you know what I mean.

I love you so much I'm afraid when I don't feel your presence. I'm afraid when you go to help others; you won't come back to me.

I know I'm selfish and jealousy runs through my body for wanting you all to myself; so please forgive me for getting out of line and don't punish me this time.

I guess I'll have to share you, like sharing a pie, but I'll still pretend; it's just you and I.

What story will your life tell today, will it be one for others to follow or will it display a detour sign?

And You Thought You Had It Bad

Excuse me, but where have you been the last couple of years?
Haven't you watched the news and seen all the tears.

Haven't you seen the pain, suffering and the devouring of
life, that's a common occurrence in our daily activities? And
you thought you had it bad.

Haven't you seen what goes on in our churches by the ones
who abuse our trust, and then have the nerves to ask us,
what's all the fuss?

I guess you don't see all the lives being lost by those who
paid the ultimate cost.
And you thought you had it bad.

Let's not forget about the cities and islands we go to for
relaxation and peace of mind, no one thought they would be
going there to see how many dead bodies they could find.
And you thought you had it bad.

Do I need to say more or have you gotten the picture? That
look on your face tells me selfishness is one of your traits, so
I better continue before it's too late.

Mudslides in the west; hurricanes in the south and don't
forget the kids that are starving because they have nothing
to put in their mouth. And you thought you had it bad.

What about those parents, who bury the ones that are
supposed to bury them. Have you walked in darkness like
the blind, knowing there is no switch to bring light into your
world? And you thought you had it bad.

Have you noticed the faces on the posters of the missing?
Didn't they tell you someone in church went through what
you're going through or even worse and they survived?
What you should be; is thankful, because you're still alive.
But you still think you have it bad.

Have you sold your children into slavery or prostitution,
because you thought that was the only solution? And you
thought you had it bad.

Maybe this will drive it home. The next time you want to
complain because you think you have it bad, just imagine
you being in the coffin and it's your family, that's sad.

Dreaming

I've sailed the seven seas, flew to the moon and even ran with cheetahs in the jungles of Africa. I've soared high above the clouds with eagles on my left and eagles on my right, descending back to earth without a care in sight.

I was a blimp gliding peacefully across the farmlands of the Midwest, while soaking up the sun's rays.

I was that fireman you saw carrying a baby out of a burning building, to the sounds of cheering fans, not for me, but what I had in my hands.

I scored the winning touchdown in a Super Bowl, and pitch a no hitter, all in the same day. I performed open heart surgery at the age of ten, at the risk of losing all my friends.

Tonight I think I'll hang out with the stars, not the ones we see on television; but the ones who shine light on us when the moon is absent.

Since I'm in the neighborhood, I might as well drop in on my other friends in the Milky Way, to visit for a while and listen to what they have to say.

I traveled with the wind as it blew across desert sands. I found a cure for Aids, with this cure, I'll save millions of lives, maybe then, we won't be afraid to shake hands and can stop covering our eyes.

Why don't you come along, it doesn't take much and it's not very far. We don't have to dress up or use your car, simply close your eyes and hold on tight, let your mind wander while in flight.

I'll even show you what's at the end of a rainbow, no one seems to find. I'll show you what lies at the bottom of that continuous fall we sometimes take in the middle of the night.

Just for coming along, I'll show you how to keep the money we hold tight in our fist, only to wake and see reality turn into a wish.

I've ice skated with polar bears at the North Pole, the only evidence of that is my frost bitten toes.

I came ashore with the high tide, being very careful not to make a mess as I tried to hide from loneliness.

I was the thorn that stuck you as you pulled a fresh rose from the bush. I later became that leaf falling gracefully to the ground as the seasons changed.

I'm that humming bird hovering in mid air as I take a pause between drinking the sweet nectar of flowers, on my daily stroll through the pasture.

At one point, I was the richest man on earth, not because of money or possessions, but what I have in my heart.

Moments later I awaken from my deep sleep, to the sound of someone screaming; then it dawned on me, I was simply dreaming.

No one ever said we had to dream small. Remember dreams do come true. So when you dream, dream big, and it's ok if your dream makes you feel like a kid.

Rainbow Chasers

Pots of gold, barrels of silver are just some of the treasures
they say lay at the end of rainbows. There are other treasures
more valuable and waiting to be discovered and you won't
need containers to put them in.

Some treasurers are so priceless, you have to go through
things to get them and they'll stay with you your entire life.
What you chose to do with them is up to you.

Some of the wealthiest people are homeless, handicap,
diseased and malnourished. They don't have the privilege
of taking life for granted. They do, however still have hope,
and sometimes your hope can be too much for you to bear,
especially when people just don't care.

We call these people "Rainbow Chasers" and their treasurers
are being healthy, being able to do things that normal people
do, like walk, talk, run, jump and see. They just want to be
like you and me.

We hold our heads high whenever we pass them by. Dirty
looks, pretending we don't see them and refusing to spare
any change, no matter how much we have, because we think
they're insane.
Could it be we're just mistaking the truth that's right in front
of us, because some people do need help? When it's time, the
Rainbow Chasers will be in the front and not in the back,
they'll be first and not last and all we have to do; is blame
our past.

Watching Mama Cry

I'm an old man now, who's been just about everywhere and seen just about everything, from disasters to death, but nothing comes close to watching mama cry.

I can't imagine doing anything that would bring mama to tears, but there are some things in life a mother deals with that's suppose to make her sad, in order for us to see an example of love, pain and happiness.

The first time I saw her crying, I was a child, and I questioned the GOD she prayed to every morning, not knowing he was my GOD also, so I vowed not to believe in any thing or any one that would make mama cry.

I learned that crying is a part healing and healing is a part of growing. The understanding comes later as our mind develops and receives knowledge, that's passed down from generation to generation.

It hurts me to this day to even visualize mama crying, so I try to avoid the nightmares at night as well as daydreaming throughout the day.

Mama sometimes confused me, like the time I brought home straight A's on my report card and she began to cry after looking at it. So dummy me replied, don't cry mama, I'll do better the next time.

That's when the smile came to let me know her tears were tears of joy, and from that point on I knew nothing was more valuable, more pleasing or more soothing than a smile on mama's face and her warm embrace.

Who Said Love Doesn't Hurt?

I thought it didn't hurt, so I never prepared for it. I was told as a child love doesn't hurt, just like they said Santa brought our presents if we were good and left him cookies and a dime, only later to find out mom got them by working overtime.

Whoever said love doesn't hurt, has never had their heart broken, has never lost a love one, has never felt rejection and has never watch their parents act as if they had money to get you gifts, knowing all along they didn't have a penny to their name, but they knew saying no, at that point and time would only bring hurt and pain.

Whoever said love doesn't hurt has never watched the dreams of their children disappear in a matter of seconds, and there was nothing you could do, other than share their emotions and the agony of their defeat that was left not only on the field, but forever in their mind.

It hurts me to know what my Lord and Savior had to endure so you and I could be where we are today. So don't tell me love doesn't hurt when I'm sitting here in tears imagining him on the cross.

If it's real, true, authentic love then you must hurt in order to feel and know just how much you love someone. For love will show itself and when it does, it's as if heaven opens up and all your blessings come at once.

If you're around long enough, you'll no doubt have your opportunity to see it at it's worst, but don't give up on it because it's been known to come around more that once.

Don't tell me love doesn't hurt, because I've seen it at its best, when they laid grandma to rest, and my entire family cried, because we knew she was on her way heaven, because her job here was complete.

My confusion was cleared later that same night when she paid me one final visit, just to say, love really doesn't hurt if you let it have its way.

"The bending of knees and interlocking of hands only tell half of the story".

The Storoem Writer

It's official, unanimous and unbelievable. I am he. I've been given the unthinkable task of taking the situations, problems, and blessings, life has given us and transform them into words.

No matter how long, difficult to pronounce or spell, no matter how big or small, they will no doubt tell all.

I've always loved to travel, but that was for my pleasure not others. I must now go to places many pray they never have to go, places that stain our hearts and minds; places that give us laughter and joy, places that bring tears to our face and make our body ache.

I have also been given the title of "The Constant Traveler", because I'm about to visit some of the deepest and darkest holes, as well as beautiful tropical islands and paradises.

You and I will cry, rejoice, hurt, be confused and misunderstood, but that's life and life's presents are not always put in our hand.

You will see hell as I see it, because he's allowed me to see it, and it may not be to your liking, but that comes with the job.

Heaven is as beautiful as one could possibly imagine. It's soothing and peaceful. There is however a fee, but you have to take that up with the boss, he sets the price, I just tell you how much it cost.

I'll be a little bias, because he's always been so good to me, so the pictures I will paint, that I have in my mind will set you free. That's if he sent you that way.

It's not too late because my assignment has yet to start, so get your life together and flush out your heart.

Remember, I'm just the Storoem Writer, when translated means life's stories in the form of poems, and I can only write what you've done or didn't do, so good luck and may GOD bless you.

A Little Bit of GOD!

It's a great way to live your life, so I applaud you. How can one go wrong by putting a little bit of him in everything they do?

It's like putting flour in a cake, sugar in Kool-aid; the more you use the bigger and sweeter it gets.

Relationships are filled with him, but we never know it's his love until we're away from them.

Many put him in everything they cook, especially around the holidays, just so you can compliment them, when they look.

A little bit of him can and will go a long way and that's all you need to complete your day.

It should start the very moment you open your eyes in the morning and last until you close them at night.

It gives you this feeling you can't describe, so don't waste your time trying, no one will believe you, and they'll probably think you're lying.

Grandmother showed it to mother, and mom showed it to us. All we have to do is believe and give him our trust.

It's just fine if you put a teensy, weensy bit of him into your life, because a little is better than none at all, for without him you're sure to take a fall.

Being Tough

You mean to tell me after all these years of building up
my body, just to have it torn down was all for nothing.
And you ask me, what's the reason for the frown?

I abused my body by starving it, drying it out, not to
mention polluting it with all types of pills, and now you
tell me that stuff kills.

So how am I going to get tough, build muscles of mass
and on occasion, talk a little trash? Being tough has
nothing to do with how much you can lift or bend or
impress your friends.

Being tough doesn't come from the appearance you
display or how much time you spend in the gym.

Haven't you heard that it's "Not the dog in the fight, but
the fight in the dog", what do you think they meant, by
saying that?

Let me explain. Being tough is a state of mind and if
you haven't exercised that, then you're wasting your
time.

Toughness shows up when you least expect it, when
you're cornered and you have no where else to go, but
straight and through whatever it is or was, that got you
to this point.

So don't flex your muscles the next time someone wants
to know if you're tough, because you may be showing
them how weak you are.

Just be quiet and let them figure it out on their own and never let anyone knock you off your throne.

The Wooden Floors

They've been replaced by musicians, bands, choirs and televisions. I guess that's a start, but they'll always have a place in heart.

Some of the magic's gone, but not forgotten. The healing power and cold chills we received, when they talked to our souls, let us know we're never alone.

It's sad to say, we only remember them with the loss of love ones. That's what happened to me as I sat in the pews and listened to their rhythmic stomps without music.

That's when the child in me returned and I felt like I was nine years old. At that very moment I knew I was back where I belonged, back home.

They creep when we walked throughout the church, some spots were hollow, and others had boards extending through them, which made a distinctive sound and let everyone know you were in a particular area of the church.

There's something heavenly about those floors, they speak to us when words just won't do.

As a child we laughed at the old women who stomped so hard their panty hoses came down around their ankles. We didn't know better, but mom explained it later, verbally and physically.

Silence often filled the air as the sound of someone walking, echoed through the walls, but we never saw anyone. That's when the wooden floors let us know he was there.

We sat up straight, pretended to be paying attention, so our
names wouldn't be mentioned. If that happened we knew
something would be sore later that evening.

I still love those wooden floors and the magic they possess,
and I hope their around when it's time for me to rest.

A Forbidden Place

What had taken twenty years to build quickly disappeared with raising of a hand, and at that moment, that second, that hour, that day, my dreams became obsolete and a thing of the past.

In a matter of seconds my life and the elements it took to destroy it, flashed before my very eyes and I knew what lay ahead, I'm afraid to say, could cripple me and possibly take me to my death bed.

Now I must fight what I've allowed to come in and disrupt my life, and no one has to tell me, I have to make things right. How, is the missing piece of the puzzle that has to be found and molded into place, and soon, if I want to stay in this race.

I don't know if I'm entitled to dream again after the way I handled the last one, but I'll ask anyway and hope he listens to my side of the story. It's worth a try, even if I did bring him dissatisfaction instead of glory.

What was I thinking when I put my hand in the place it's forbidden to go. So now the masquerade is over and it's time for the real show. What came over me, what evil did I let in, it surly wasn't me, because I'd never hurt my best friend.

I always said it would never happen to me, no matter how bad times get, as if I knew this day was coming. Only Prophets can do that and I definitely know I'm not one.

So forgiveness is in order, starting with myself, and it has to be believable, genuine, not on the outside, but inside where it really matters or I'll become one of the many that's scattered.

*The heart can travel to places-
the mind can only dream about.*

The Butterfly Parade

I've past this field on numerous occasions, smiling as I watched them flapping their colorful wings that make me want to sing, but I know I can't carry a tune. So I continue smiling and absorbing the peace I see them enjoying.

I promised myself, one day I would join them, so I too can bring smiles, laughter and joy to someone who's had a rough day, like they do for me.

As I watch them synchronize and become one entity. I can only imagine the sense of freedom and the beauty of togetherness that fills their heart.

With their antennas transmitting the sweet sound of the language they only understand. The field becomes one giant display of love, and it engulfs the rough day I thought I had, and let me know my day wasn't so bad.

Tomorrow I'll join their ranks and become a float they'll have to hold, so I don't fly away and miss my chance to feel freedom.

Even if it's for a brief moment, I'll still thank GOD for another wonderful day he made, and for allowing me to become a part of **The Butterfly Parade**.

B.I.D.

Everyone's saying I should be happy and smiling from ear to ear. I don't see what they see, but it's kind of odd so much good is happening to me.

It's said if you're looking for them, you'll never see them coming. They blend in with life's situations, so you may or may not understand what just happen or how it happened.

You thought you were just lucky, because things were going your way. You thought you were in the right place at the right time. How far from the truth you are?

They come when we least expect them, majority of the time we don't deserve them, but that's how he operates.

Some times we go around questioning ourselves with questions like, Was that one, I'm sure that was one, I know that didn't just happen?

When we know we've done something wrong, we have the nerves to say I've been blessed or my prayers were answered.

Let's set the record straight, those were not your prayers being answered, but the prayers of someone who knew you wouldn't pray yourself and they knew you needed help, because sinners need prayers too.

Some never realize what happened until it's too late, but that's their fault as well as their mistake.

Then there are those who receive them and still go around mopping and don't realize they've had a good day, not to mention the dreams they let slip away.

Blessings shouldn't hurt, at least some of them. Sometimes they have no choice but to bring you to your knees, because you forgot the magic word, Please!

They're called **B**lessings **I**n **D**isguise and they're supposed to make you wise.

Tongue Tied

Out of the blue it attacks you and there's no remedy
for it. It either let's you know you've meet your soul
mate or lets others know you're lying.

It happens at a moment's notice without giving you
any prep time, so what comes out, you can only hope it
doesn't make you look like a fool.

Letting mothers know you did something you weren't
suppose to, tells fathers to get the belt ready, if you're
a son. Being "tongue tied" at times, is no fun.

Some encounter it with the anticipation of love or a
brush with death. Known for making you forget your
name, for saying words out of order, not to mention
your sentences make no sense.

Your tongue isn't really tied in a knot, but there are
times you wish it was. It sometimes sound as if you're
speaking a foreign language, when that happens there's
always a friend to make you feel like a clown.

I believe it was invented to remind us we're human and
mistakes do happen and if nothing else, it lets us know
we need to slow down and not always be on the run,
because in life everyone should have a little fun.

Holy Water

It's used to warn off vampires, if you believe in the old folk tales and movies on television. Pleasing, soothing and fulfilling are just a few of the words we use to describe it.

Depending on its direction of travel, let's everyone know what you're going through, but they still may not be able to help you.

It has the power to clean the stained windows we call eyes, when you're too confused to see a little house cleaning needs to be done.

It's known for flushing out the soul and removing the weight you really don't have to carry. It reduces pain for a while and allows you to show your beautiful smile.

I've seen it make people laugh and cry, scream and holler, run, jump and bend like rubber bands, but that's what comes with the laying on of hands.

Most waters are tasteless and have no color, but Holy Water is beautiful to see and refreshing to the body. It's a small taste of heaven, when it's taking out the trash you've kept in the house to long. It simply makes you strong.

Holy Water mends broken hearts, soothes the pain of losing a love one, quenches the thirst for understanding, restores joy and the abundance of life and erases all of our fears, and it's just another name we call, Tears.

Peace Therapy

Today is the day I've dreaded would come, but I knew it
would, sooner or later. Now I have to open up and let them
enter my world, my secret garden and sacred shrine, not
because I want to but it's what the doctor ordered.

I really don't know why I have to go see them. Maybe it's the
mood swings or nightmares or could it be the depression
that has me going to my first session.

As I entered the room, it seems they were prepared for me
and anything I could throw at them. Their first words to me
were, have a seat on the couch, sit back, relax and kick off
your shoes, we're going to be here a while".

They let me start off, by describing my symptoms. My reply
was; I don't have any, because I don't need to be here.

One of them decided to start by saying let us have your keys,
we want to be your friend and friends don't let friends drive
dazed and confused.

As a matter of fact, this session is free, because there's a lot of
work to do, we see it, why can't you?

Tears will be shed and that's just fine, it helps to get things
off your mind. You won't cry alone, because we'll share your
pain with you, not to deceive you, but that's just what we do.

We're here to get you back on the right track and we'll do
whatever it takes. There's enough lost sheep's wandering
around, without adding you to the number of the lost and
found.

So we'll see you next week, this is just a start; our ultimate goal is to repair your heart. It won't happen over night and you'll definitely have to fight, especially if you want what's yours.

No one said peace was free or you wouldn't have to pay a price, just how much are you willing to pay; is the question you'll have to ask yourself. How much will it take to clean up your mistake?

"GOD is good, all the time; all the time, GOD is good".

When it comes from the Heart

We have only to thank society for some of the mess we get ourselves into, because we're willing to claim; by speaking, and accept; by acknowledging, the illness, pains, failures, corruptions, and many more negative situation in our lives.

Why do we go around allowing our mind to put us in uncomfortable situations we really don't have to be in?

I'll tell you why. It's because we listen to our minds sometimes and not our hearts. Our hearts are pure and without hurt and pain, until we start listening to our minds. If your mind hasn't been cleansed, developed and nurtured, then you may be in for a lot of trouble.

The heart can take us to places; the mind can only dream about, places the mind can only think about; places the mind's afraid to visit.

It's like writing; those who write because they have to, will never reach their full potential, because the mind can and will only take them so far and to certain places.

But the heart, oh my, when it comes from the heart, your writing is unlimited, passionate, loving, endearing, healing, soothing and needed. It cannot lie, no matter how you try to cover it up.

The heart can bring you to your knees if it has to, hopefully you'll be able to thank it and have learned your lesson, because it doesn't give you too many sessions.

One Day I'll be Happy

One day I'll be happy and I'll owe it all to you. I'll smile again and this time it won't be a fake one. I'll show all thirty-two and it'll be from ear to ear.

My struggle will be over and my joy will return like a breath of fresh air on a warm spring morning, like the smell of honeysuckles that leads bees to paradise.

There will be no more walking while intoxicated with life's problems, no more being afraid to share myself as if I was a leper. No more being afraid to talk about topics that made me cry inside and fall to the floor as soon as I opened my door.

I've lived a life of lies and deceit to myself, family and friends, but now I see the poison as I sweat profusely and my blood pressure skyrockets to the point of exploding.

This is the life I've selected after being given the opportunity to be selective. I was blind, but my eyes were open, deaf, but my ears were clogged, speechless, but my voice remained silent, tired, but full of energy, depressed but full of joy, lonely, but full of memories.

I've had good days, great ones too, but I didn't enjoy them because I forgot about you. Planning vacations and imagining what a wonderful time I would have, often got my motor running, but I remained in park.

Eager to be adventurous and see the world, but my eagerness has also crippled me with the intention of spoiling my dreams. I'll be happy again one day and all the treasures I've missed along the way, they'll still be there waiting for me to pay; attention and respect to those who sacrifice a piece of them so I could be happy once again.

I said I'll be happy again one day, so don't worry about me and the things I say. Simply make room and place another plate on the table, because I plan on joining the rest of you, just as soon as I'm able to.

Who's Helping Who?

So you thought you were helping others, you thought what you were doing would help and benefit them. When are you going to open your eyes and take the blinders off?

It's obvious you haven't looked in the mirror lately and seen yourself. You haven't realized why you've been so tired and have no energy, but that's what denial does, blinds you.

It covers your pain, you forget your name and how to smile and this is just the first mile of this race they call life.

You forgot one important fact of life; you forgot about you, you stopped taking care of you. It took for an old friend to come back in your life, just to tell you what you didn't know, to show you what you didn't see.

Miraculously, you made it this far, how, I'm not sure. You call yourself a writer, and you just knew you were writing to share your blessing with others, and to help them rebuild their life, to let them know their life isn't over because of a few problems.

You were so busy thinking you were helping others, you didn't notice the hurt and pain in your own life. Remember when everyone kept asking you how you were doing, how was your day going. You thought they were just being polite and courteous.

No, they saw what you thought you were covering up, what you fail to see and didn't want to believe. A battered man at the end of his rope, a weak and fragile body crumbling like old news paper.

Not knowing how to ask for help almost brought you to your doom. But it's ok; it's a new beginning, the first day of your new life. It's time to let the past, pass. Don't let anyone or anything take away your joy or dictate how you go through the coming days.

Let go of that bag of weights you've been carrying around with you, that has made you age, that has made a young man reach for his rocking chair before his time.

You thought you were helping others; I believe others were helping you. Life has given you a new start, time to make a few decisions, to put the pep back in you step and while you're at it, don't forget to say thank-you. With that being said; what are you going to do?

A Talk with My Friend

The last time we were together we walked side by side, mesmerized by the understanding of that moment. You with the level of my confusion and me with the depth of your love.

This time I think it's fitting that we pull up those two chairs we talked about. I'll do the listening and this time I won't let any distractions filtrate my mind.

It's been a while, at times I didn't know if I was going or coming, if I was growing or shrinking. I ask myself, did I wait too long to ask for assistance, by listening to my mind and not my heart?

Your presence is a welcome addition to the company that I've sat at the table with elaborating on subjects and issues we were unfamiliar with.

Now that they've seen me with you, that smile on their faces lets me know they need you just as much as I do.

It stills amazes me the amount of satisfaction and strength you give to so many with just the thought of your arrival. But, isn't that what true friends do, sit and listen when you pour your heart out, when no one else wants to.

Teaching My Brother

I later found out it was part of his teaching and not because he didn't love me. It was the beginning of many classes he would teach.

Why aren't you helping me was the look I gave him, but he continued to watch until I figured it out and realized I would have to do my part, before any assistance would be given.

He never told me it hurt him as much as it hurt me, but I saw it on his face, I just didn't know what it was. The discipline it took for him not to get involved is something I'm still searching for.

There were times when we didn't see things eye to eye and we had our little scrimmages. I knew then, like I know now, he let me get a few punches in to build my confidence.

I've always thought he was invincible; others did too, so he was rarely challenged. He never went looking for trouble but when it came, he stood up, strong, and proud. He held his ground and let no one push him around. I will always admire him for that.

Sundays in the park were an adventure. I can still see him pulling on the basketball rim. I never said it, but I was always happy he allowed me to hang out with him.

He told some of the funniest jokes I've ever heard, sometimes they didn't make any sense, but they were from him, so that didn't matter. I was just thrilled to be in his company.

Bus rides to school, as painful as they were, I'm glad they were brief. I saw it on his face, through that fake smile we made, like it didn't hurt. But I know it hurt him, like it hurt me.

If I could go back and relive those days, I would ask GOD to exchange my laughter for his pain, my accomplishments for his disappointments.

I just want him to know I love him to death, if there is such a thing. He made me the richest brother in the world and I'm glad GOD gave mommy him, and not another girl.

Dedicated to Barney (Red) Thompson, My in the middle brother!

The key to future blessings is what we do today.

There is a difference between Poor and Po!

Many use it as a punch line to their jokes never having a clue to the difference between the two. They often offend those who've lived it, like me and you. Maybe this quick history lesson will shed some light for those who can't get it right.

If you're sensitive and have compassion in your heart, I don't mean to make you cry, but when I'm finish there won't be a dry eye, and that's after mentioning the ones that only hurt a little.

Let's start with having one roll of toilet paper compared to the rubbing of newspaper together so you don't scar yourself after reading the headlines.

What about when your bathroom door won't close compared to your bathroom being outside, we called them outhouses.

How about having a blown light bulb instead of a candle for your lights? And you didn't know there was a difference. Pay close attention, there are a few more I didn't mention.

Don't forget telling your brother not to mess up his clothes because they'll be your wardrobe for next year. Just the thought of that is enough to bring a tear, but you didn't get upset because you knew that was the best that could be done.

I remember when it was time to move and I waited for the moving trucks to arrive; and there they were right on time, my brother and sister pushing four buggies.

Let's not forget a trip to the hospital which meant a visit to grandma's medicine cabinet; the real hospital.

What about some of the dinners we had which consisted of the cheapest meat in the frozen section, topped off with noodles or maybe some rice, with all types of seasoning, they call it gourmet these days.

We washed that down with real kool-aid, better known as sweet or sugar water. If we wanted dessert, we had to wear belts made of snickers, if you know what I mean. And you didn't know there was a difference between Poor and Po.

Now their wearing Jordan's and Iverson's costing three digit figures. We were lucky if we got a pair of Slip and Slides or Bo-Bo's, and that was with the help of selling old bottles or cans.

Air conditioning was sleeping with the window open in the summer and having it cracked in the winter. That's because we didn't have to worry about crime, like we do today. These day's kids have rooms to themselves with signs telling you not to enter. We were happy if we had enough room with girls on one side and the boys on the other.

Sometimes during the winter, we were called Michelin man, because of the layers of clothes we wore compared to the kids with new coats. That went along with the nickname of "Clown" for having shoes filled with stuffed socks because the shoes were too big, but we eventually grew into them.

How many times did you hear that? Believe me when I say it isn't a joke, just the facts. I wouldn't trade them for anything, because it taught me the real meaning of family.

Do you still believe there was no difference between Poor and Po? If that wasn't embarrassing enough, try going to a friend's birthday party and your gift was whatever you could find to put in a brown paper bag.

And yet, we were the richest family in the neighborhood. There is no amount of money that could replace the smiles and laughter we shared together and that's something we'll have forever.

Now you know there really is a difference between Poor and Po. When someone tries to explain it to you, tell them you already know.

The Protectors

They came to the rescue every time the alarm was sound; never knowing the cause or what they were about to get into, but whatever it was, it wasn't enough to deter them from coming.

It was obvious to me at a very young age that blood is thicker than water.
The sight of them riding in on their white horses always brought a smile to my face, because I knew I would soon be safe.

I was always teased about them the following day. If my friends only knew the sense of security that came with them being my protectors, their jokes would've turned into applauses.

They answered every S.O.S that went out and I knew they would, so I had no doubt. Why is it, as kids we don't express our feelings for the ones we love?

Let it be known now and forever more, to my protectors I say this, I love you more than you could ever imagine.

You help raise me to become who I am today. When others look at me I hope they see the beauty of you in me. You taught me about the birds and bees as we sat and talk underneath the mulberry trees.

Yes it's true, you were my protectors and I'm sorry I didn't tell you before, but one of these days, when I make it big, I hope you know I couldn't have made it without you nor would I have wanted to.

My Protectors; My Sisters, Helen, Beatrice and Charlie Mae.

When Did You Know?

Why do you beat yourself down, knowing eventually it'll get better? It's ok to hold onto that little bit of hope. But remember, sometimes we all have to play the role of the dope.

The first indication was, when they didn't smile like they use to after making eye contact. That's when I knew things had changed.

The perking of lips followed by a kiss, was a scene that diminished too three maybe four times in the spanned of a week. What a drop off from five to ten times a day.

When we no longer finished each others sentences or enjoyed a movie together, it never dawned on me; maybe it wasn't supposed to last forever.

The laughter had stopped along with the compliments and opening of doors. Those things didn't have the same affect they used to.

The hugs didn't feel the same, because you can feel love in an embrace, and see it on their face. You were in denial and couldn't believe someone had taken your place.

Remember dressing alike and the looks that came with it? Whatever happened to those days, where did they go? That light at the end of the tunnel is no longer clear; maybe it's trying to tell you the end is near.

You stopped doing what it took to get them, so the attention came from someone else. You used to get away with the fake smiles that covered your pain, but now it's external and your picture is worth a thousand words.

Was it when you entered the room while they were on the phone talking in codes. It had to be codes because you knew they didn't speak a second language? The interlocking of fingers while holding hands, had become a thing of the past.

Just maybe it was when they insisted on going to the mailbox after telling you, you've had a rough day, just relax; became an evening slogan.

It could have been when you went on your walks that used to be side by side, now it's one in the front or one in the back. Was it when I Love You converted back to a simple "Me Too"?

It's not the end of the world as you can see. You can always start over, but leave the past in the past. Now it's time to grab hold of your future and maybe this time, the laughter and love will last.

Facing Your Demons

It has become and will continue to be an uphill climb and constant battle, if you don't face them head on or before they get too strong and cast doubt, fear and illusions, that's really not there, while you're in this weaken state of mind.

They're in control of what you thought was yours to keep, what you thought was free of charge and came with no strings attached, but you're finding out the hard way, not everything is a perfect match.

To enjoy peace, freedom and paradise, one has to endure some type of pain, get knocked down, kicked around and learned how to crawl, before you take that ride down the golden highway.

This is just the beginning of what lies ahead, to see if you're worthy of staying in his presence, because he's always waiting for us to do our part. He'll never leave you alone, don't you know that's how he earned his seat next to the throne.

You've given your demons too much respect, too much power and now you're confused as we approach that hour. Do you go this way or that way, up or down, around, over or through what's really not there, you would see, if you would only stop and stare.

One by one they'll begin to fall, just stay in his presence and give it your all. When the smoke has cleared, the tears have dried and the hurting has stopped; the laughter will return, stand and be strong, lift your hands and let everyone see your victory dance.

Putting it in His Hands

You've tried it your way, and it's not a surprise things didn't turn out right. Every time the outcome is different, maybe you should try using another name, and this time hopefully you won't be the one left holding onto the pain.

You've read all the books and it seems everyone has their own way of dealing with life, but you don't deal with life, you live it.

So why are you so empty? With the smell of peace in the air, but you're all alone with no one to care for or about. There's no one to share your happiness and love with and there's still a little doubt.

Will he help you, if he loves you or if you're worthy of ringing his doorbell and ask to come in; out of the rain and shame, you've brought to his name.

Forgiveness, a word rarely used by someone whose pride has made them look like a fool, knowing all along, their grief was, is and won't go away, until you put all of it in his hands.

You have to let go of the past, the pain, the hurt and the things that have kept you in bondage. It's simple and plain to see, all you have to do is listen to me and put it in his hands, so you too can be free.

I hope you get the picture and won't be the jerk that doesn't move on, even though you know the victory has already been won.

It should be easy to shake that tree you call your body and watch the dead leaves that have kept you locked in your cell, that made your foundation tremble like an earthquake; fall to the ground.

Once that is done, and only then, will you receive that breath of fresh air and be able to embrace love and the other gifts that come from above.

"You will never get relief,
if you never release".

Convincing Yourself

You feel bad and you should, what you did, made a lot of people sad. All you had to do was walk away and keep your mouth closed. But no, you had to prove you were a man or woman and disrupt your quality of life.

Doors are being slammed and you're sitting in the dark, all because you just had to leave your mark. Afraid to walk by mirrors because you know what you'll see, something you were not meant to be.

Now your conscience is constantly beating you down, it's taking advantage of this opportunity, because it doesn't come very often. You've given it another chance to mold and sculptor a weak and fragile soul.

Your apology has begun and it starts with you, forgiving yourself. It does no good to apologize to others if the source is still evil and hasn't been cleansed.

You have to be sincere and true to yourself, if you're to convince those you've offended, so they'll believe your anger really has ended.

If you don't except or believe your apology is real, what makes you think anyone else will. So apologize to yourself, for you, and make it very clear, because no one should have to go through life living in fear.

Humble Me, Lord

Unable to complete such an easy task, I've allowed the anger within to hold me hostage and prevent me from enjoying the spices of life.

Help is needed now, so I'm placing my call to the one who sees and knows all. Hopefully I haven't waited too late and he doesn't have too much on his plate.

The question no doubt will be asked, why didn't I do it myself? Simply put, I have nothing else left. After the stress and unwanted guest, now I'm down on my knees Lord, asking you to clean up my mess.

Forever in debt, but this is one I'm more than happy to repay. Nothing in this world is free, so I'll give you my heart as collateral until my mind and body catches up with me.

I'm asking you to humble me Lord. I know I failed to comply with your instructions on how to get by. Another chance is what I'm asking for and this time I won't live a lie.

Please humble me Lord; I swear I've learned my lesson. I promise I'll never abuse another blessin.

Down Home Cooking

So you had to go where it all started and mix the ingredients together again. You lost your character and forgot who you were. Its pay up time and you're down on your luck and don't even have a dime.

You made more enemies than friends, so you don't trust anyone and have no one to turn to. I guess now would be a good time to get on your knees and pray until your face turns blue.
As you began to fill your pot with the missing ingredients, be sure to add a little bit of "forgiveness", followed by a pinch of "I'm sorry" a table spoon of "It won't happen again". That should be enough to get you a few friends.

Don't feel bad because you're not by yourself, many of us put ourselves too high on the trophy shelf.

So now you need some "Down Home Cooking" because your life is a mess and you didn't stay grounded, so you failed the test.

Be thankful we have a forgiving GOD who loves us, answers our calls and picks us up after we fall.

Now you're back where you belong and hopefully you've learned your lesson and know that not every day is promised to us.

Don't forget to count yours the next time you have a chance to brighten some ones day, remember, just like they're given they can easily be taken away.

Crying Without Tears

An element of my life I've mastered without anyone knowing; one I'm not proud of because of the ultimate price I'll pay one day.

I knowingly assisted in the terminating of my own life, not by choice, oh no, by my incapability of letting go of bad love, love that devours my existence minute by minute.

Afraid to let my tears accompany my cry, so they contaminate the fluids that slowly evaporate and take a part of my spirit with them.

The toughness I display does no more than eat my life away. I'm tired of running, but the tears won't come, and I've tried so hard, but the puddles that use to clean my system are on the blink.

For now, I'll prepare a statement that will one day explain my fall and how I let bad love take my all.

The professionals call it "Dry Eyes" or "Desert Eyes", but all they know is it describes a situation when our cries go unseen.

They may be unseen but not unheard, whether it's crying like a baby or taking a stand after your pain can no longer be tolerated.

A cry is what you'll produce in one form or another, with or without tears and it may last a brief moment or a few years.

The sound of your voice cracks no matter how long you hold your tears back, and those who really know you, come to your aid because they know it's not good for your health and one day it could be the source of your death.

So pray when your cry comes, your river flows south and help tell your story with the help of your mouth.

Making Love

If you think it's just a physical thing then you haven't experienced its true meaning. Making love is continuous; it's up to you to bring it into your life.

Making love starts the moment you open your eyes in the morning until you close them at night.

For me is seeing that smile on your face because I know it's for me. It's holding your hand as we walk through life together. It's looking into your eyes and seeing how much you love me.

Making love is giving you a massage after a hard days work, it's you laying your head on my chest until you fall a sleep, and wake up and I'm still there holding you, that's making love to me.

It's running my hands through your hair and hearing you tell me how good it feels. It's seeing how proud you are after the struggles you had to go through to get where you are today.

Making love is what I do when I look at your face when you're sound asleep and don't know you're smiling. It's what I do when I'm driving home, knowing your face will be the first one I see when the door slowly opens.

It's also what I do when I kiss your feet and watch your toes curl from the sensation you get as my lips make contact with your skin. It's what I do every time I tell you, I love you.

Making love is the foreplay that prepares you for the intimacy that comes with the connecting of two bodies. It's what I do from sun up to sun down and whenever you're not around.

Making love to you is a dream come true and it's all I ever wanted to do.

Crisis is not the time to lose your faith;
it's the time to believe in your faith.

The Cotton Field

They stand side by side, one behind the other, all moving in unison. What a dazzling display of happiness and fulfillment, for brightening up someone's life.

Every time one is plucked, one is replaced, so there's never a shortage. They protect us from cold in the winter, heat in the summer and loneliness in the dark.

They surround us when the enemy is knocking at the door asking to come in when they know their not allowed and can only come in, if invited.

When the wind blows I see ruffles of white waves, pleasant to the eye, magnificent in spirit and soothing to the soul.

Floating in mid air; all dressed in white constantly letting you know everything will be alright.

The Cotton Field is replenished with the dying of the flesh and birth of eternity. No more weights to carry as your burden is lifted.

It's time to rest as your purpose in life is revealed to you and you become one of the many bushes of cotton wanting to be plucked, so that you too can make someone smile or someone's dream come true, like all **Angels** do, now that you're one too.

The Sound of Music

What could be more pleasing to hear than the sound of music in my ear? Once you've heard it I'm sure you will be amazed, how the sound of music puts me in a daze.

It makes me laugh, it makes me cry; it makes me smile like a rainbow in the sky. When I'm sometimes down, it picks me up and when I'm at a high it has brought me to a low. That sweet sound of music really makes me go.

I feel so complete when it's around. Oh how I love that sweet, sweet sound.
The sound I love, that's so dear to my heart, is my companion's voice that tears me apart.

She's the twinkle in my eye, the pounding in my chest, that's how I know I have really found the best. If you ever meet her, I'm sure you will agree; that sweet sound of music could only be _____.

Blind Man Walking

How can it be explained, do I even try, but tell me, how does someone that can see continues to walk around running into everything that gets in their way.

Unable to see what's not seen because of a cloudy mind, so you delay your blessings that wait in line.

Constantly coming to the wrong conclusion because you don't want to believe what has happened, so the blinders you're wearing prevent your advancement in status and stature.

Blind man, blind man; open your eyes so the things you bump into won't be a surprise. It's ok to feel bad, but the worst thing you can do is get mad.

You feel the pain while you stand in the rain, but there's no shame because you're not the blame. Your eyesight can be corrected with a little time and patience, so can your flight.

Don't let your mind be your guide, listen to your heart, it won't steer you wrong, it will build up your immune system and that will make you strong.

Your prescription was filled a long time ago but you were too busy, now you're the show. The use of a cane to assist you when walking has become your mode of travel.

It didn't have to be that way, if you had only listened and given your life a little time to unravel. Then next time you call yourself cleaning house, make sure you don't forget to clean your windows.

Alone, But Not Lonely

As the photo albums come to life and tell the stories I've lived, I find myself traveling back in time to places that brought smiles and happiness to a very shy child.

Even the pictures on the walls find time to reminisce as they recall the lighter side of a life filled with joyful memories.

Yes, I am alone, but far from being lonely. How can one consider himself alone after living what some would say is the "fullness of joy"?

Lonely is being in the presence of no one, it's when you have no recollection of happiness, which is something my life is filled with.

As I put into motion a new beginning, I look forward to a future that brings the best out of me, a future that allows me to live out my fairy tales and dreams.

I invite you to come along and share this passion I have for life. Together we'll experience the luxury of friendship and the dominance of love that's sent from above.

If I have nothing else, I have the stories grandmother told, that alone is enough to keep me out of the cold.

There will be others awaiting our arrival with open arms, a sight I've longed for. I don't want to disappoint them and I plan not to. So the invitation stands, now the rest is up to you.

The next time you find yourself standing in a room and think you're alone, try closing your eyes and let the darkness take you home.

Dazed and Confused

What do I have to do, is the question that now confronts me; it's also a question I can't answer. It would be and should be easy, if not for the torture I put myself through.

By doing that, I call my father a liar, a title that is unfitting and undeserving for my king, but that's the message I send to those who come in contact with me.

Frosting on the outside, as sweet as I want to be, but that along with my blessings are washed away as moonlight turns to day.

Dissatisfaction is the word I'm sure he uses when asked about me, I know he doesn't want to give up on me, but what word could be more defining, more describing to what you see?

He's done so much for me, is it because he thinks I can still be saved or he knows my life is slowing crashing like a tidal wave? Sympathy is what comes to mine, and I'm glad he gives it out from time to time.

I've dug a hole too deep to get out of, was given enough rope to hang myself, burnt too many bridges to get back to the other side, so now I have nowhere to run to and nowhere to hide.

I've been given all I need to stop this madness and pain, but that too evaporates, like falling rain. The answer is clear, but I've chosen not to hear, maybe that's why the answer remains unclear.

It's as easy as A, B, C and 1, 2, 3, all I have to do is ask for a little help and do my part, that's normally a very good start.

So I guess the question wasn't hard after all, I should just be thankful for the blessings I've been given or prepare for a fall.

Enjoy
      Life
           Or
              Endure
                    it.

Because of You

I wouldn't be who I am nor do what I do, if it hadn't been for you.
Thank you is in store and well deserved, and I promise to be there
for you like you were there for me.

Because of you Mother, my heart is soft and tender, you showed me
sacrifice with a smile and that I'll always remember.

Because of you Father, I'm strong and firm, something you have to
be when raising a family, so the kids will learn.

Let me take this time to acknowledge those who I'll forget, because
the list is long and I don't want anyone to get upset.

Because of you Sister, mother is never far away. You're a reflection
of her and that's how I'll always see you. You taught me the
meaning of protection and to never let anything stand in my way.

Now Brother, you have to know, because of you I spread my wings
and go, you showed me freedom and in return I just thought you
should know.

Because of you Aunts and Uncles, I know mother's life wasn't
boring. I listened to the stories when you sat and talked, so I could
tell them, when we take our walk.

Because of you Cousins, I knew help was always there, when it
seemed no one would listen or cared. You taught me to keep change
in my pocket just in case I had to make that call, so you could come
running to my rescue and I wouldn't take that fall.

Because of you Nieces and Nephews, I learned how to take care of
children before it was time to leave the home and have children of
my own.

Because of you Daughter, I can stretch out my arms and become a blanket of love; you showed how the simple things, such as a smile, can be so precious to one's life.

Because of you Son, I was taught the true meaning of being proud and that there will come a day when we'll have to let go of our childhood.

Because of you Friend, I know family can come from places other than mom and dad.

Because of you Love, I know how I got here and why I'm never alone, why I should appreciate the little things in life and be thankful for every day and every night, and because of you Love, I know GOD.

Because of you GOD, I know all of the above, and if not for your love, there would be no above. Because of you, I cherish each breathe I take and the mistakes I make.

Because of you GOD, I hear the birds sing and see the joy they bring, and I know it's all "because of you".

Her Sacrifice

I made it my job to help her relax anyway I could, so I had my tools ready, because she knew I understood. You would be amazed what a comb and brush can do to someone who's given their all.

As I began to scratch her head while she sat on the floor, after a hard days work, she began to tell me how her day went, but I knew because she seldom made it to her bedroom.

She slowly began to drift off to sleep, which was another sign she had spent too much time on her feet. Too young to know what I was doing, by reciting poems in my head, I later understood what I was doing was and is called praying.

She never said how tired she was or complained about the hours she had to put in to keep food on the table. There was no need anyway, because I knew as I untied her shoes and by the sigh she made after they were removed.

As time passed and her shoulders began to slouch and her speech became impaired, her tone lowered with every breath she took.

That was one picture the dictionary painted for me, only it was in words. Nevertheless, it brought a smile to my face because I felt the love as my fingers ran through her hair.

Such a powerful act of sacrifice being displayed not only at my home but right in my arms, one that benefited me when I got out on my own.

As I sit here with tears in my eyes and try to do the unthinkable, of trying to tell her how much I love her, sacrifice is trying to tell me it wasn't all it seemed. I'm not listening because I feel the sacrifice every time I give her a hug.

I didn't know it at the time, but sacrifice has a way of playing with your mind. It tells you no one appreciates your hard work and effort you've made to keep things running smooth, and then it reminds you the bills still have to be paid.

She would manage to get a few hours of rest, because that's all you're allowed when raising a family by yourself. If I could have, I would have lifted the burden she carried around for so many years, but then I would've missed the example and definition of sacrifice that now brings me to tears.

Now that I've seen sacrifice at it's worst and its best, I realize it's just another phase we go through before we can rest. One of these days I'm going to bring a smile to her face like she does for me, as I help her sit in what I call, the recliner of life, so she can relax until GOD calls up his next group of angels.

Love you, Mommy!!!!!!!!

Tell-Tale Signs

A good example of "in bad shape" is what I am, because of the disease that pollutes my mind and body. Constantly being asked to play the man in the red suit, at Christmas time because of the depression that's being stored below these broad shoulders of mine that no one wants to lean on anymore.

The inability to lose weigh; after starving myself with diets and countless hours in a gym puzzles me. All of this could have been avoided if I had only listened to him. Now walls are closing in, along with shortness of breathe and meaningless conversations with myself, is just a mere test that I fail over and over again, no wonder I have no one to call my friend.

Mommy said there would be days like this when seconds seem like minutes, minutes like hours, hours like days and you walk around in a daze. Could it be these are warning signs I've overlooked and my failure to recognize them is all it took; for bedlam and mayhem to come into my life.

I've been told there's a remedy that camouflages the signs and lessens the pain until I recover and remove the stains, so I don't live the rest of my life in vain. I have yet to come across it so my afflictions continue for the moment. I refuse to give in or give up until these stained glass windows, I call eyes, are cleaned and I can see the light that's promised, if I can endure this fight.

State of Confusion

So happy, but yet so sad; so good, but yet so bad, tired of being tired of being constantly mad. What am I to do when it seems nothing I do brings joy and laughter?
Misery has me for company, so it needs no one else. You can pack up your worries and cares and place them on the shelf.

I'm confused and now I have to play this game, win or lose things definitely won't be the same. That's acceptable because it takes away some of my pain.
Dense fog and cloudy days prevent me from feeling the sun's blistering rays. Even the stars hide as the night swallows me whole and consumes everything I have, including this tired and battered soul.

The faith I thought I had is no where to be found, and falling to my knees won't help either, because my voice refuses to make a sound.

Pretending to be bold and strong, pretending to be made of steel, pretending nothings wrong, pretending, pretending, and pretending.

My thoughts are few and misunderstood to say the lease, but I must continue in order to have peace.

Traveling by foot has slowed as if I'm wearing concrete shoes. The weight of my world has shifted from my shoulders to my feet and what was once too heavy to carry, now makes it harder for me to move forward.

I've learned that confusion is really a state of mind that we put ourselves in when we're out of line. It's a plague that devours the good times we could have had, but we settled for the scraps and now our happy has become our sad.

Life's a puzzle and my pieces don't fit, but I have too much to look forward to, so I definitely, can not, will not and must not quit.

Why Me, Lord?

Could it be, is it possible, you've made your first mistake by selecting me? Questioning your decision is something I would never do, but I'm confused because I know I'm not worthy of speaking to you.

The errors I continue to make, lead me to think I wouldn't amount to anything, now you come back into my life and tell me I'm something.

I guess it's true when they say sinners need you too. After all I've done and all my fun, you still think I'm worth saving.

Am I a statue that needed to be polished for its value to be seen? Have you removed all the makeup that hid the beautiful creature I believe you created me to be?

I know there's a catch Lord, so what do I have to give you this time. It can't be much because I'm pretty sure I have nothing you can use or need.

I think I know what I can give you to make you smile and be proud of me again. What if I give you my heart, my trust and simply believe in you, would that be enough to make amends?

So the question is no longer "Why me, Lord" but "Why not me, Lord"?

"A little bit of GOD, goes a long way".

6 x 9

Alone in my cell with no one to talk to, no one to see
but these walls that have stopped my advancement,
my development and my growth.

Is this why my days have become longer and my nights
shorter? Is this my punishment, to live within these
borders?

I find myself alone and isolated from the human race
and sentenced to my doom. I've made up my mind
that I'll fight to the finish, however long that may be.

One day these walls will fall and my freedom will be at
hand, and only then will I be able to make a stand.

I've lived in my 6 x 9 long enough without knowing the
reason. Is this what my life has come to? Is this what I
leave as my legacy, not if I have something to do with
it?

So spread the word that I'm on my way and nothings
going to stop me, at least not today. I've limited myself
to the straps off the table like a dog that's lost his bone,
not to mention I don't even have a place to call my
home.

My space seems to diminish as my 6 x 9 continues to
shrink, which leaves little room to insert my thoughts, my
feelings and my desires, all because I took the advice
of one or two liars.

So let this be a lesson learned and not a lesson earned,
because there's still time before the jury adjourns.

When Your Home Becomes a House

Someone made a mistake and twisted my world around. As I inserted my key into the door of what's suppose to be my castle, a place where you should always have peace.

I find myself in need of a "divine intervention" because my home has become a "how to survive" convention.

The smell of candles used to greet me at the door, but that too has been replaced with an unpleasant odor.

Is this what I'm to grow old with, as my days become few and numbered? Am I to give in or put up a fight, just so I can make things right.

I built this house from the ground up, brick by brick, frame by frame, so why am I afraid to enter my own domain.

One would think that they would at least be able to sit on their own throne, but that's what happens when your house is no longer a home.

Afraid to cook and clean, but this is your house, so what do you mean, you're afraid to cook and clean, or answer your own phone. You're right; your house is no longer a home.

When She's Not There

If you haven't done it, then you haven't been in love, not just any kind of love, but deep love. How do you know it's the real thing and if she's the one you want to wear your ring?

It's simple, and you can't hide or fight it, some don't even realize they're doing it. Doing what you ask? Doing things that you did together, but this time she's not there.

You go to the restaurant and order dinner for two, when it's just you. Play her favorite song and play it all day long, these are just some of the things you do when she's not there.

You even watch so call girlie movies at certain times of the day, because you know she would be there lying in your arms.

When you lay down for the night, you spray her side of the bed with her favorite perfume; drift off to sleep hoping she'll be back soon.

You think about your first date and how you made sure you wouldn't be late. The first time you cooked for her, while walking around in your birthday suit. Not to mention you cook dinner for two and set the table as if she'll be there too.

And you thought only ladies did things like that. As your day passes and you walk around with that smile on your face, it lets everyone know your body is here but your mind is in another place.

Don't be ashamed, you're not alone and there are others who care. Just remember, these are just some of the things men do, when she's not there.

My Two Friends

Never get tricked into answering which one you love the
most, either love them the same or plead the fifth to save
yourself the pain.

They're always fussing and fighting, neither thinks they're
ever wrong, so I wind up playing the middle man, just so
they won't get out of hand.
One's nice, the other's mean, ones good, the other is bad. One
sits on the left the other on the right. That's one way I keep
them separated so they won't fight.

One gets me in trouble, the other gets me out. There's a soft
side embedded in one, while the other has a mean streak that
keeps unwanted visitors away.

When I'm angry, one feeds fuel to the fire that's deep within
me, while the other one extinguishes it when he knows I've
gone far enough.

They're like night and day, one stays with me when I get in
trouble the other runs away. Why not just get rid of the bad
one, you ask. That's because it's a two package deal. You can't
have one without the other, so don't even bother.

One you definitely want in the heat of battle and the other
you'll need afterwards to tend the wounds and mend the
scars. Yes, these are my two friends and I know they'll be
with me until the end, that's what true friends do.

One refuses to take the blame for anything when he's given
me bad advice, by saying he didn't tell me to do that, I did it
on my own.

One believes in dealing with only the facts, while the other lives for rumor control.

One's proud of me when I achieve a goal while the other downplays the struggle I had to go through to get where I am, as if it was nothing.

There will come a day when they will have to split and I'll have to decide who will stay and who'll have to go, right now I really don't know.

With friends like these two, I don't have time for enemies and if I did, I probably wouldn't know what to do.

Waiting on the Son

As I take my morning walk on the beach, I feel so alone, because my friend isn't here and he won't be until this darkness is gone.

So for now, I'll continue to walk and count the minutes as they pass, because I know this loneliness won't last.

Sometimes he's a little late and that's understandable, on other days he doesn't show up until late in the evening and that's just to check and see if I'm where I should be.

He's a good listener, and he knows some of my darkest secrets, and I know he won't tell and that's another reason we get along so well.

When I take a step, he takes a step, when I turn around, he's somehow on the opposite side, and I don't think he's trying to hide only staying with me stride for stride.

What a true friend he has turned out to be, he makes me so happy and I'm comfortable when he's around and I hope he never leaves me.

Tomorrow I'll check the weather forecast, so I'll know, the exact time to expect my friend, the one I call, my shadow.

Some people will never read a bible,
but they will look at your life.

The Price of Peace

What I thought was free of charge now has a price tag on it.
How and what you will pay depends on how bad you want
it, how bad you need it, if you deserve it and what you're
willing to go through to get it.

The type of currency you'll have to pay may not come in the
form of paper and pocket change definitely won't get it.

Some say blood, sweat and tears should be enough to get it,
the old fashion way, but if Satan has anything to do with it;
he'll try to have the last say.

It may cost you more than others, sometimes it's less, but
that's only if you've been at your best.

Are you willing to endure long term suffering, isolation from
family members or are you one of those whose looking for
a handout, sorry to say peace doesn't come with a payment
plan, but you will pay, the question is what?

It's well earned if you've lived your life right, but there will
be times you'll have to put up a fight.

An accomplishment some never achieve until their death,
why wait so long, when it's yours to have why living, all you
have to do is follow a few simple rules, because that's what
life is, a continuation of schools.

An arm here a leg there and if you're really lucky, you'll only
get a scar. Peace has never been free and if anyone can testify
to that, it's me.

Don't give up on it because you'll do yourself a great injustice, allow yourself to go through the process, because you don't want to miss out on this.

The Pause

I'm there and it's not by choice. The decisions I've made and the company I've kept, while walking around with my eyes closed, got me there a little faster than I thought it would, and now it's time to take a back seat and have a second look.

Everyone has a pause; the secret is how you deal with it once you get there. How long you stay is determined by the level of understanding you have upon your arrival.

While in the pause certain things will be revealed and certain things will be healed. Being afraid to let go, afraid to accept what's happened, what will happen, just extends your stay because you're in need of nutrition before you get away.

Time won't stand still but you certainly will, as you try to sort out the mess you're in. There's no need to call your friend, because when he tried to help you, you didn't want to listen.

You will walk, talk and look the same, but you won't be the same. Those who know you will be amazed after your transformation has taken place. You'll even have doubt yourself, why this stoppage has occurred. Your past has been wiped out and if you're smart you'll let it remain there.

How did you get here? It could have been a number of things, your job, a friend or a lover that has brought you to your pause. Sometimes it takes a date with the devil to open your eyes, in some cases a slap in the face is all that's needed to get you in the right place.

Let's hope the time you spend in your "Pause" is short, nutritious and a step forward for you receiving your wishes.

Sh, or You Might Miss It

Where did that sound come from, who decided that it
needed to be made? My eyes don't see what is definitely
commanding silence.
An authority figure, no doubt, because I feel its presence and
it's caring a lot of clout.
Sh, it tells me once again, if I want to witness the signs,
miracles and wonders that display themselves on a daily
bases.
Sh, if you want to hear the angels surrounding you to deliver
the protection that you will need as your enemies try to deny
you what is rightfully yours.
Sh, if you want to see love and how it sooths and calm the
savage beast and the lonely at heart, but first you'll have to
do your part.
Sh, if you are to learn the lesson of forgiveness that you will
need in order to be forgiven.
Sh, if you want to feel the affection others have for you for
what you've done one time or another that brought smiles to
their faces.
Sh, if you are to teach what you've been taught, whether
it was good or bad, it happened for a reason, just like the
changing of the seasons.
No, you don't get the chance to say anything; you no longer
have that right. So here's a tip, just sit back and keep a zipped
lip.
You had the chance as you lived your life day after day. That
was your time to make a difference, to author your own
book, to direct your movie. So for now watch and learn and
hope you get another turn.
Some say you learn more simply by being quiet, if that's true,
where's my degree, because I've sat in silence long enough.

Sh, you're doing it again; elaborating on something you don't understand, why else would they tell you to put it in his hands?

Sh, for the very last time, or you'll definitely miss what I have been sent here to tell you.

By the way, my name is Holy Spirit, I don't normally make house calls, but this one was needed, because you are definitely headed for a fall.

What Have You Done?

You've started something new before you ended something old, and now it's not only your life that's in shambles or just your story being told.

Never meaning to hurt anyone was your intention, but you let this get away and out of hand. Now your answer to those you affected is, I don't understand.

Refreshing a damaged soul is not an occupation one chooses to put on a resume, because damaged souls need to be healed or repaired not refreshed.

Your heart is not the only one that needs mending because of the mixed signals you've been sending.

Bringing pain and old wounds back into someone's life seems to be your trademark that's left every time you depart.

Nightmares are revisited, so sleep is deprived of someone's well deserved rest, but it won't come today because of another fine mess.

You thought about yourself and didn't realize the destruction that followed you, and once again you've made someone else's life blue.

Giving hope to someone is a gift, snatching it back within five seconds would confuse even the strong at heart, but that's what you did right from the start.

What do you have to say for yourself after the humiliation you've brought to the family name, are you sorry or simply the blame.

Just look at what you've done. I'm ashamed and can't believe this is coming from one of my father's sons.

Friends Don't Do That

If it was me, I wouldn't listen to him after all the hurt and pain you've been through. How could you even think about someone who's brought you to your knees, not to mention he took your prize possessions?

I thought you were my friend, how could you say things like that knowing how I feel about him. Those things you call prize possessions, can't go with me, if I want to ascend on that cloud when it's time to go.

It's obvious you've heard the stories and didn't understand them, so let me shed some light and give you a little insight. There's nothing you can   say or do to make me stray.

And you call yourself my friend. Friends stand by your side when times get hard, comfort you when you've been left standing in the dark. That's what friends do. I thought you were one too.

You want me to end the relationship I have with him, because of what someone thinks or believes. What a waste of your time, not to mention mine.

I think you woke up on the wrong side of the bed and the devil has put nonsense in your head. Friends don't do things that calls you to get your mouth washed out with soap and let others know you're really a dope.

They do however; stand by your side when times get hard, comfort you when it seems your life is falling apart. They hold your hand when you're traveling down that lonely highway and let you know everything will be OK.

That's what true friends do; I guess I was wrong, because I thought you were one too.

"Don't cut your life short by wishing your days away".

Now You Know

The instance it happened, I knew we were destined to be together, and this time the feeling told me it would last forever. As we made eye contact, I felt your soul, and I knew there was no turning back.

My heart took over and it guided me forward, toward what I had searched the world for, never knowing you were right at my front door.

Now you've entered my dreams and I don't want to be awakened. It would be too painful if I'm mistaken. You held my hand at one of my darkest hours, and we conquered my fear together.

Your grip was like no other as it gave me security. It was gentle as a flower, but strong enough for a man.

What we've been through in our past, has prepared us for our future. What lies ahead, I'm not sure, but I'm not afraid, because you're with me now, and our dues have been paid.

Our souls connected and now both of our lives have been affected. I tried love before and had to put up a fight, but something tells me this time, I got it right.

GOD at my head and you at my feet; standing on top of our world with the feeling that my life is finally complete.

Happiless

Its how I've chosen to live my life, because it is a choice, but not many make the decision I did. It doesn't have to be this way, but it's one of many tests that lie in the path I must now travel if I'm to ever rest.

Not wanting to be around anyone and no one wanting to be around me. Why would anyone want to be in the company of someone who turns picnics into funerals with their mopping around and an upside down smile on their face?

I soak up everyone's happiness like a wet sponge constantly being rung out in order to make room for more. Feeling bad is something I can do by myself, but you know the old saying "misery loves company", so I try to steal as much joy as I can before I'm called to leave this land.

Asking to be rescued from this great gift I've been given puzzles me. If I would only take the time to evaluate what I'm giving up on, I would probably realize how easy it is to go from happiless to happiness.

I've cried wolf one time too many and it seems my luck has run out. No one's paying attention to the drama they're use to seeing whenever I'm around, because they're tired of me bringing their high down.

I'm on my own now at least that's what I thought, until an angel whispered in my ear telling me it's not over yet, this is just one of my falls, he'll still listen, all I have to do, is get up and make that call.

Wearing Handcuffs

It didn't have to be this way nor did it have to be the day
your decision making comes to an end.
Now your language is filled with regrets, should haves and a
few too many apologies.
You've relinquished the gift of doing it your way and now
your hands are tied behind your back.
There's nothing you can do because it's his way now, and
that's a fact.
No more dictating your life scene for scene, you abused that
privileged as well, and now its time for a new routine.
Why do so many chose, not to leave well-enough alone, is it
that they're greedy, selfish and constantly wanting more. Not
once do they take time to look at the score.
One life for free filled with unlimited happiness and joy, all
you had to do was to follow a few simple rules.
Getting out of order is a major set back, one that will cost you
more than you can afford. But that's the path you've chosen.
Now history will repeat itself and it has you to thank,
because your life can no longer be annoyed.
Being told what to do, how and when to do it is something
you're not accustom to.
Now you're about to learn that freedom is not free at all,
everyone has to pay a price before they get that call.
We'll save you a little embarrassment and won't give you a
number to go with your new orange suit, you've earned that
much for trying a time or two.
Not in control anymore and there's no one to intervene,
you're going to have to sweat this one out, so go ahead and
kick and scream.
Your handcuffs may be loosened, but removed, I think not.
That's the price you have to pay for losing control, so now it's
your life that's on the clock.

The Sweet Smell of Morning

A conformation that lets me know a new day has begun with the rising of the morning sun. So elated I've been allowed to witness beauty at the start of my day, I fall to my knees and began to pray.

As I open up the house to let it breathe, I'm greeted by the aroma of the awakening, they too have a reason to celebrate and it's obvious as I listen to them serenade the gift of life.

What an intoxicating smell that penetrates the sensors in my nose and gives me a lift as I rejoice at the sight of the morning rituals carried out by a number of species, including myself, who can't wait to see what the day has to offer.

Such a desirable smell served with the birds singing, squirrels playing in the trees and butterflies spreading their wings in preparation for their morning flights.

How can I not be thankful for such a breath taking sight and it would be selfish of me to even think of not sharing this with others, so that is a lost thought.

As the flowers unfold their landing strips for the bees to begin their work, I am reminded of the partnership it takes to spread this type of enjoyment around the world.

Lasting for only a few hours each morning, I know its time well spent, so tomorrow I'll be in the same place, same spot waiting patiently to be mesmerized before the day gets hot.

You Asked For It

You begged, pleaded, prayed and on occasion demanded.
Now that it's been given, you say you don't know what to do
with it.

It wasn't yours to ask for, but you thought you deserved it,
so you constantly bothered your father, for the attention you
didn't need.

You're like a new born baby that just left its mother's womb
and sees the world with its own eyes for the first time.

Do I look this way or that way, do I touch this or leave it be,
but you can't because there's so much for you to see.

Words are spoken to you for the first time in a language
you've never heard, so you think it's just noise.

Your understanding will come later, because you rung the
doorbell too soon and asked for help that wasn't needed.

Your life was good, but it seems you never got the whole
picture, so the meaning wasn't understood.

Walking in the wilderness can be a delight, if it's done right
or it could be a long and treacherous trip, if your mind is not
equipped.

Fine tuning is what needs to be done, but you're not ready if
you're still on the run.

You've missed blessing after blessing and hindered a few,
because you didn't step out on faith and that's the reason for
the mistakes.

The load you bare is of your own doing, so you have to marinate in it for a while to get the message.

Smiling faces and the shaking of hands awaits your arrival, because they went through the same process and they know how you feel, when you don't understand.

When you dream, dream big;
even if it makes you feel like a kid.

When Loneliness Creeps In

Like fog coming off the ocean it works its way in without
detection. Its goal is to make you as miserable as possible.
In a room filled with people, but yet your mood swings go
unnoticed by everyone but you, the victim.

One moment you're sky high, the next you're down in the
dumps. Why the change as if you don't already know. This is
one battle loneliness must not win or the out come could be
your end.

It can't creep in if there is no invitation, so don't plan
the occasion, do what you have to do even if it means
participating in meaningless conversations; because it's the
company you need, not the discussion.

If allowed, it will steal your joy, a forbidden feat that must be
avoided at all cost. The decision has to be made to fight; and
when you fight let it be with every ounce of your strength.

No need to worry because this story is only the beginning,
and loneliness has crept into a place where it has no friends.

The walls have closed in and it can not breathe; my
suggestion is that it packs its bags and leave. But, if it won't,
there's a remedy for that as well, I've read some people call it
hell.

If loneliness is still determined to stick around, no problem
let it know that smile on its face will soon be a frown.

Is It Possible

Is it possible for me to love you the way I do after being gone
for so long? Is it possible that my words will come together as
I try to sing your song?

Is it possible this fear I have of you being the one
I've searched the world for, keeps me from making a
commitment to you or is it just the excuse I use for not
saying, I do?

Everything I've ever wanted in a woman I see in you, so
why am I still feeling blue? Why do I get nervous with the
thought of us being together and at the same time get excited
about the possibility of holding your hand, these things I just
don't understand.

You've always been special, that you never have to prove.
Being in your presence is enough for anyone to realize the
angel you are.
Now that I've found you, please say you'll stay, so that my
search doesn't have to continue another day.

Is it possible what we felt for each other in our past still
remains, and if so, how will we know? What a beautiful sight
you are to see, one that I dream of waking up every morning
and find laying next to me.

Is it possible that what I'm trying to say will one day come
true and you'll love as much as I love you?

Undecided

Unable to make up my mind, so I sit alone in my world
questioning myself. Was I quiet when I should have spoken,
did I speak when silence was required?

Thinking everyone would wait until I made up my mind
was a bad call, now my back is up against the wall

Indecisiveness has infiltrated my mind and cast doubt in my
thoughts; it has cost me many treasures and much grief.

I'm punished it seems for the path I've chosen to travel, so
I travel it alone. Must I now live my life in vain to diminish
my pain?

The answer is no, but it took a friend to show me the light
and let me know life is too short and it must go on.

If I had made the decision when the opportunity presented
itself, if I had listened to my heart maybe my new beginning
would have already started.

When you're hurt and confused, the right thing to do seems
to be the wrong thing to do. I've procrastinated so long it's
even harder to convince myself that I'm ready to make that
decision.

One will be made, either I'll do it or life will draw the line, I
just hope I'm on the right side.

Forward or backward, up or down, the decision is mine, do
I choose to be happy or sad, do I have faith of doubt or will I
do like so many others and simply let time run out.

Present, Present

Without question it's a gift beyond measure, one to die for. To understand you have to be spiritually grounded, at least it would help to be.

A gift you don't have to wait until Christmas to receive, if you simply believe. Known for being wrapped in the finest linen from head to toe and white as can be, like fresh snow.

With the exchanging of gifts, others enjoy the warmth I celebrate all day long knowing this gift is mine.

No longer does he have to raise his hand when attendance is taken because he's been acknowledged physically with the closing of eyes, mentally with the thoughts that travel through my mind.

Yes, he's present like the wind blowing across my face, like the whispers in an old house letting someone know life was once in this place.

Like fine wine he only gets better with time. What he gives and how he gives it, is simply divine.

He's a present when he's present and even more valuable when he's not. That's how I know the faith I have is more than enough to get me through this life that can sometimes be so tough.

The meaning is clear, except the present whether it's missing or present, far or near; except it with open arms and you won't have to live in fear.

Spring Forward, Don't Fall Back

It's the leap of a lifetime, one that is well deserved. You did what you had to do, now let the whole world see the new you.

After what you've been through, and having survived, is a major accomplishment and you should be proud of yourself. Not many make it and get the chance to tell their story.

It made you a better person, that's obvious to see; now you have to stay focused, since you made it here. There's no turning back let's make that clear.

Your face lights up and we see the glow a mile away. No words are needed, just continue to smile, so others can see you, and try to emulate your style.

You're an example now, so stand tall and be proud, now it's easy to pick you out in the middle of the crowd. It's alright to look back every now and then, let it be a reminder, so you don't go through it again.

The charade is over, so no more pretending to be happy when you're down in the dumps or trying to hide your scars and lumps.

Those things are no longer a part of your life, so lock the door and throw away the key. Life comes with a price, as you can see, so remember not all things in life are free.

"Let your honor outweigh your honors".

In the Midst of my Storm

The prediction calls for cloudy and gloomy skies with a
slight chance of misunderstanding.

I've prolonged a life without happiness; no wonder my aging
process increased three times the normal rate.

I experienced highs and lows, ups and downs. I experienced
the joy of happiness as well as suffering and death.

Countless days of mourning, followed by weeks of
celebrating, and this was just the early stages of my storm.

But, in the mist of it all, my friend stood tall and by my side,
even on the occasions when I wanted to fall.

The idea of giving up crossed my mind time after time,
but a part of me refused to give in because it knew I hadn't
reached my purpose in life.

The gathering of storm clouds began to form like a puzzle
being put together, and what had confused me started to
make sense.

Painfully I let my life take its course and I remained silent,
sometimes hoping and praying it would all come to an end.

But those thoughts were of a person who didn't realize they
had been blessed beyond measure.

I knew at that moment, I had been given a gift and no matter
how bad my storm would get, I had to survive and not waste
such an important and valuable gift.

In the mist of my storm I was challenged and tested to the best of my abilities. Sometimes it led to smiles, sometimes to tears, and when life really got bad, my storm even covered my fears.

Time to get out of the storm now that I've weathered the confusion it presented, and let it know I refuse to live that life another minute.

The Fool Effect

You brought it into the equation and now you have no clue how to solve the problem. One thing for certain, sitting around feeling blue isn't going to help you. Up until now, you thought nothing could stop you, you thought you were invincible, but you used the wrong formula to build up your ego.

To make matters worse, you mixed the wrong ingredients together trying to come up with a remedy to ease your pain. That's when the "Fool Effect" came into your life. Now you're afraid to go outside because you think everyone is laughing at you.

While going through the "Fool Effect", you will need help, but you won't ask for it, because you don't want anyone to know what you're going through. You're wasting your time, because it makes you act out of character, so your friends will now, but won't say a word.

The "Fool Effect" magnifies your insecurity with yourself while slowly destroying your body from the inside out. You trust no one, even those who are trying to help you. It makes you see mirages as if you were in the desert; it isolates you when you're surrounded by a crowd of people, who pay no attention to you as they go about their daily activities.

You're barely able to see the road while driving around town, because you slouch down in your seat hoping no one sees you. Legend has it everyone plays a fool sometimes you just happen to be next in line. To make a long story short, curiosity killed the cat, if you're not careful you too will whine up on your back.

Broken Glass Memories

If you have them, here is a word of advice, let them go or
they could be the cause of a break down or even your death.
One hasn't been recorded, but they have been known to take
you to the edge of insanity, which in most cases is all some of
us need.

BGM is what they're called by those who've lived with
them and can't let them go. Known to interrupt dreams,
crack foundations and devour goals; with sustained painful
thoughts and dehumanizing events.

Masters of masquerade by letting you think for a brief
moment you've made it through the worst, then out of the
blue they suck that ounce of hope you thought you had.
Before you know it you're back at square one, and believe me
that's no fun.

Failure to continue to read could turn out to be a big mistake
and if you have soft skin, then I suggest you call a friend.
They make the hairs on the back of your neck stand up, but
don't worry it won't last long; it's just an attempt to numb
your emotions so you don't relax too long.

I didn't know much about them until my mirror broke and
pieces of my life scattered over the floor. I guess I had to
experience them in order to tell our stories the way they
should be told and to warn those who still have a chance to
avoid this long and painful journey.

I've felt what falling apart feels like, I've ridden the horse
called Broken Spirit and lived a life without joy. But, that
wasn't the end of my world, just preparation for the task at
hand, to give back what I've been given; Hope.

My "Broken Glass Memories" had stripped me of everything I had except my hope. Little did I know, Hope, was all I needed.

Hope gave me another chance, hope gave me strength, hope resuscitated my body, and it brought me in out of the rain. Hope let me know I had a purpose and that's when I reassembled, glued and molded a broken heart. That's when I knew my "Broken Glass Memories" had to be put back together and this time cleaned, so I could reach my purpose and help you see yours.

GOD Is Good, Even When I'm Bad

Living in the gutter and eating the straps of this world. I was all alone until he threw me a bone not because I wanted it; because he knew I needed it. I guess it's true what they say about him being good all the times.

Have I waited too long, has my time ran out. I'm asking him for mercy and another chance. How can I repay him for something I know I don't deserve? So if the answer is no, I understand.

I made this bed now I must lay in it. I have tried my best and at times succeeded on many occasions to abuse this gift of life he's given me. I know I'm unworthy, that's why I'm so amazed at the amount of love he's shown me.

I remember as far back as a child, always seeking the easy way out, short cuts, doing the wrongs instead of the rights. How can it be, that someone who has constantly been in the wrong place at the wrong time their entire life, be awarded the benefits of the righteous, if not for his love.

Once again you've shown yourself to be good knowing I've been bad. Even crooks acknowledge you with regret, the least I can do is not neglect this second chance I've been given.

So I bow now, which is customary for someone who's come to grip, now that their equipped, with the knowledge and understanding that it's never too late, as long as there's life left in your body, to start over and hopefully I'll get it right this time now that I know;

"GOD is good, all the time; all the time, GOD is good",
even when I'm bad.

A Good Day

Waking to the sound of beauty as the birds serenade the
rising sun, I too see the beauty of this event that lets me
know we've been blessed again, so I join in and praise this
gift.

As the day continues to unfold, there are fewer distractions
in my way, so I'm able to focus on the things that really
matter and not those I have no control of.

There's calmness in the atmosphere, no sirens or gun shots
ringing out. Yes, today is a good day and it seems life has
something on its mind, something it wants to say.

With my eyes wide open and my ears tuned in, I become a
new born baby anxiously waiting to absorb what life has to
offer free of charge.

There's laughter instead of crying surrounding me, and the
vibes I receive reminds me of happier times. Yes, today is a
good day.

Blue skies filled with white cotton slowly riding on the waves
of wind followed by the smell of peace. I ask you, what could
be more relaxing? Yes, today is a good day.

As I drive these lonely highways, I realize I haven't passed a
homeless person or even a cardboard community, no signs of
graffiti or gang members on every corner and no make shift
cross that indicates the location of a lost love one. Yes, today
is a good day.

The sight of families gathering for a picnic in the park; is a glance at yesterday that melts my heart. As daylight turns to darkness, I am greeted at the door with "I miss you" there's nothing more for me to say except, today is a good day.

Now at the pentacle of my day, I must conclude it on my knees before I lay, to thank him, because today was truly "A Good Day"

A father's failure; a child's reward.

Suppose To Be Here

Echoed in the halls of my mind constantly by myself and others, I started questioning my existence. Caught up in the midst of what I thought was a storm, I failed to see the importance of what I was going through. Could it be I was being prepared for something I'm not ready for?

Realizing it was time to change my way of thinking, time to stop spending countless hours of beating myself down and injecting a dose of doubt, which I know can't be healthy.

I'm continuing a cycle that uses the phrase "I know I shouldn't be here" as if all the mirrors in my house are broken. By doing that I slowly drift away from the blessings that hibernate until I figure out I'm still here and stop telling myself I'm not suppose to be here.

Yes, my eyes were closed to the events that had kept life in such a fragile body that at one point I was ready to give in. But that's when it happened, just as I was ready to give in, reality took a stand, because I felt less than a man.

Knowing my potential it grabbed me by the hand and let me know self pity was no longer in demand. Unable to share the same establishment, the greater devoured the lesser and what you see now is what should have been displayed a long time ago.

There's no more doubting or questioning what is so very clear, even after all the mistakes, I know I'm suppose to be here.

Sometimes One Has To Endure

As I called out, I answered myself, as the sound of my voice bounced off the walls of what was a happy home.

It tells me my services are no longer needed and if I don't leave now, the ankle bracelets I wear will never be removed.

So I think its best that I pack my bags because a journey is needed. A journey I thought I had taken until it led me to this asylum I call home.

To a cave I secretly enter as the sun surrenders to the chill of the night. Not just any cave, but the cave many hermits subject themselves to when love has betrayed them.

For now, I must endure the isolation and depression I volunteered for by living in denial.

Family and friends witness this transformation from a once happy, energetic, loving person who now struggles to place one foot in front of the other.

One would think the end was near, but thanks to someone's prayers being answered, my end became my beginning and I slowly regained the strength and durability that so many was accustomed to seeing.

I owe it all to a voice I hadn't heard since childhood. The same voice that guided me on a course to happiness, a course I somehow had managed to slowly drift away from, as time passed.

The same voice that gave me the feeling of security as I laid on its floor one hot summer day.

Now I feel I'm capable of withstanding the darts life throws at me. One by one they began to fall off this patched up soul that demands to blossom with the freedom of a butterfly.

Not only does my life began to surrender the pain and confusion that prevented me from reaping the benefits I've earned for trying so hard to be the best person I could be.

It also confirms that bad things happen to good people and no one is exempt from the lessons of life. So, remember there will come a time when we all have to deal with strife.

One Stone, Two Hearts

Never intended to break two hearts, never meant to tear us apart. Never thought the mirror I looked into to see an example of happiness would shatter, but I did.

Once it was thrown, it couldn't be taken back, so I prepared myself for the cracking of a foundation that had never shown me that it could be moved.

The pain in my chest quickly grasped my attention, the buckling of the knees prevented me from taking another step, and it seems I needed more help.

The stone that came out of nowhere, disrupted a relationship that up until now, had never been tested, but tested it was, and for the first time each heart had to get strength from each other, rather than one from the other.

After making contact I realized the level of destruction this stone had caused and I knew I had to be strong, but deep down inside I knew something was wrong, because I was a thousand miles away and I still heard it moan.

It was help I found as I closed my eyes and began to cry, a cry without tears, a spoken cry, a cry that one does when the pain is too much to bear and the load is too heavy to carry.

This too I knew would pass, because heart ache, heartbreak and hard times don't always last.

Self-Inflicted Wound

Eyes open, hearing intact as I lay in my comatose state of mind. Able to hear it all, but yet they talk as if I'm not here or can't hear them.

They're calling in a specialist so I must be in terrible shape. As I look around the room, it reminds me of a jungle filled with vines and ropes.

They continue to prep me until he makes his entrance. Now the drawing begins as they outline my chest with dotted lines, to make the incision process easy.

Not a moment later he enters the room, gliding across the floor, with tools in hand. With a quick glance at my x-rays, he states my problem; a massive amount of dead tissues caused by neglect, misunderstanding and forgiveness.

My actions have led them to believe that I asked for, what is a certain death. Unable to speak or move, I pray that the water that fills my eyes overflow and the tears somehow grab their attention and say what I can't say, "I'm Sorry".

To have made it this far is a mystery that goes unexplained. The question now becomes how they repair or should they repair the damage, if I'm going to refuse to let go and forgive what happened in the past.

Everyone deserves a second chance, so I hope someone says yes, but if not, I think I better blink my eyes a few times to speed up the flow of tears.

Suddenly out of the blue an unseen voice comes to the rescue. It whispers softly, but with authority, and the work begins.

To say I'm thankful, would be out of line, instead I'll offer my heart and pray I don't go through this a second time, because I would probably lose my mind.

Paradise

Times sure have changed and not for the best. What was once known as the Ghetto's penthouse is a thing of the past. As children we thought it was paradise, one of God's gifts from above.

Cookouts followed by house parties that ended when the neighborhood bullies decided to go home, because no one would dare tell them it was time to leave, or until your parents pulled the plug on the record player.

If there was a fee to enter, it was normally paid with the bringing of a pot luck item. Laughter rung out from every corner of the house. Conversations had many topics, filled with lies, as we talked about each others outfits and who we would go home with later or kissed before the climatic conclusion, which was the "Soul Train" line and a slow dance with the one you had your eye on the entire night.

This was paradise for many of us as we left our communities from all over town.

For a period of time, we left our worries and concerns behind. Mom and dad would walk in and check on us periodically and then back to their room, closing the door, as if that would mute some of the noise.

You were lucky if they didn't come out and cut a step or two. If that happened, it was the talk of the school for a few weeks, but that was a part of paradise that usually meant we had a good time, it also meant we weren't ready to let go of that piece of paradise, no matter how short, because it was ours and at that moment in time, nothing else mattered.

One + One = One

(Fact or Fiction)

My Kryptonite

No longer known as the man of steel, too many have seen me in my weakened state. Showered with bullets in the form of insults, misunderstanding and cruel words that use to bounce off the surface of my brain, now penetrate my skin deep into my vein, which shows a side of me that was well hidden in a solitude place in the back of my mind.

I was once the destruction of a hurricane, the fire of a volcano and had the will to withstand the coldness of the North Pole, but yet I was as gentle as a kitten with the grace of a ballerina, as soft as clouds floating across the sky, so why am I barely getting by.

There are times when I lock it up and throw away the key, not realizing it's there to protect people like you and me. Needing to see results in order to believe showed my immaturity and the lack of trust and it's just another foolish mistake I made along the way.

Could that be the reason it doesn't answer when I call for help in such trying times or am I to continue this voyage blind? The feeling of being unworthy and not entitled to be in its presence is a feeling that has lingered in the air a little too long, so I have to find another way to be strong.

Apologizing is the cheap way out, but it's a start. My downward plunge started soon after and there were no hands to grab or bars to hold on to, when there should have been. Yes, I have lost one of my friends.

There has to be a solution, a cure, at least a pain reliever, because I can't keep this up. My kryptonite, it seems doesn't come in a physical form, so it won't be seen, but you can bet there will be a price to pay for losing "My Faith".

Shelf-Esteem

Down in the dumps and having no one to thank but
yourself. Now you're allowing others to break you down.
Dusting off the furniture, moving pictures aside to make
room, as if you're receiving an award.

You've placed your self-esteem on the shelf with all of your
other what-knots, a place where it doesn't belong. You'll get
your award but it won't be one for the shelf. This award
comes complete with counseling and therapy.

Not by request, but demand, and yes you ordered it without
even knowing. Accepting fault for mishaps by other people,
defeat before the battle is won, giving up instead of getting
up. So go ahead and clear that space, but if I were you I
would do a quick trace.

Go back to where your downward plunge began and that
will tell you who your true friends are, it will show you
who's at fault. It will remind you what made you happy, what
made you smile, since it's been a while.

There you will find the answers to how you get peace,
love and happiness back in your life. It's time you start the
process of rebuilding you and closing the gap between what
has interrupted your passage from one realm to the next.

Glorious days and greener pastures wait, but you have your
work cut out for you and your journey starts by substituting
shelf-esteem with self-esteem and when this is done, maybe
you'll be able to dream.

Weeping Hour

My weeping has endured longer than a night, so my joy is no where in sight. Continuing to pray is my course of action because I know one day I'll get that satisfaction I humbly wait for.

It symbolizes new life, the new birth after letting this world go. My hope remains high as long as I keep looking towards the sky, you see, I too need help to get by.

Misery has a crowd, so tell me Lord, where do I find my peace. It's needed because I feel I'm in that hour where there's no doubt I need your power.

I know you hear me and you're always there, never late and always on time, but something's different and I'm in despair, so could you please send me a sign before I go out of my mind.

My nights are long and sleep limited trying to keep the nightmares defused to avoid a consuming explosion that's determined not to leave an ounce of life.

Within my hour I wept because of happiness, sadness and pain. I wept for sunny days as well as rain. Confusing at time, soothing for a while, but make no mistake I've walked the first mile.

The hands on the clock refuse to knock, on the door that's locked from within; so I listen to the darkness that creeps around throughout the night and lets me know I'm not alone.

I'll enjoy its company while it shares my seclusion. My hour will end soon and the weeping will stop and maybe then I'll be allowed to reach my mountain top.

The Nigger and the Klansman

Signs of ignorance best describes the use of the words, so be careful when selecting your vocabulary in your daily conversations. How dare you, try to convince yourself there's a positive side that goes with their definition.

Nevertheless, the story has to be told and if you're not soundly grounded you might get left out in the cold. I'll try my best to put it to rest and while I'm at it I might as well confess, that I too have failed this test.

He saw me standing there as he drove by in his horse and carriage, and with the tipping of his hat and the raising of my head, we acknowledged one another.

No one saw us, so our secret was safe as we entered that forbidden place. There was no reply of "yes sir, master" after being called a boy. No, this time there won't be any joy.

Having a lot of junk in the trunk or full black lips is just another way we identified each other, another was white faces painted black to let us know we were brothers.

Mixing the races together doesn't make matters better; it just leads to harsh nicknames while attending school. Half-baked and jigga- boo, just to name a few, hurt just as bad then and believe me they still do.

My white sheets lie on my bed at home, while he was wearing his as an outfit. So I wondered what type of meeting he was going to and if I would be welcome there.

As I drove around town with my flag flapping in the wind, drawing attention and getting dirty looks; I knew if they could, they would snatch it off and use it for a door mat.

So that this message hits home, don't be ashamed, you're not alone. And if that confused you, try this on for size, he's black and I'm white, surprise!

Bad Medicine

I stood to introduce myself, but the reason I'm here is already known, so there's no need to go into detail. I'm an addict who craves for the bad medicine I can not let go of.

I need help so I must attend these meetings with those who think they can relate. This medicine they say is bad for me, constantly calls my name and I'm too weak to ignore it.

Having injected myself with so much, for so long I can not quit cold turkey, and to be here talking to you today, I consider myself lucky.

It supplies me with treasures and gifts, how can it be bad when it feels so good. It has to be a mistake, a misdiagnosis on the doctor's part, so I will seek a second opinion.

Knowing it's bad is not enough to keep me away, so I find myself on bended knees, hands together, head bowed and eyes closed; the only way I know to really flush my soul and continue running this race.

At times I'm not sure I want to let go, but if I don't I'll have to answer death's call. A relapse is possible, so it's one day at a time, but it really has a hold on me.

Finding an antidote to relieve the pain is a hard and difficult road to travel, I feel I am slowly committing suicide, but that's what I asked for by not letting it go.

What was once energizing and healthy now carries me to my doom if I do not let go of it soon. Rather than continue on this downward flight, I think I will call it a night, and when I awake hopefully this bad medicine will be out of sight.

When My Struggle is Over

Rejoicing will be the theme and you'll be able to tell when you hear me shout and scream. I'll perform a victory dance because I've made it through my storm.
As the benefactor of a turbulent life, I'm rewarded with a renewed soul.

My scars have been removed and I've been given a clean bill of health. This is the beginning, after the end of a few down pours of rain and a brief moment of being insane.

So excited I don't know what to do, you would be too if you knew what I went through. When my struggle is over it'll be time for a well deserved rest, one that has been visualized time and time again, because I knew one day my storm would end.

Patience is a required taste that builds character, so when you come out of the dark there won't be any questions about the type of person you are.

When my struggle is over I'll be well on my way to securing what is rightfully mine. Satisfaction has been guaranteed, like he said it would as they nailed him in three places to save you and me.

Fresh air and blue skies travel with me where ever I go; they too celebrate now that I've cleaned my plate. Now there's room for peace, happiness and joy and that makes me feel like a child whose been given a brand new toy.

Now that my struggle is over it's easy for me to love and be loved in returned. That's all I've ever wanted, and all my heart has ever yearned.

The Seamstress

Piece by piece she stitches and repairs all the holes that can tear apart a friendship or family. Whether it's with a needle and thread or the warmth of her embrace, she's always there to console the weary at heart and those who are down to that last gasp of air that's needed to ask for another chance at forgiveness, happiness, laughter, joy and the list goes on and on.

She restores the gifts from above that so many have let slip away. She gets you back on the right path so you can receive the one's that's out there just waiting on you to get it together.

She holds whatever it is that you've lost with the nodding of her head, as she tells you, now is not the best time for you to confront those who brought pain into your life, but it is time to be proud and speechless, so they won't know that they've gotten under your skin.

I don't know what I would do if I couldn't see her face, hear her voice, feel her embrace, receive her wisdom, absorb her love or cherish the memories and moments we've shared together.

She makes you think about how many times you've been blessed and where you would be if not for the hard work of others. Why throw it all away she asks, or is it those sacrifices mean little to you.

The thoughts of her are many and the memories are plenty, Yes, I love my seamstress and the things she holds together and if nothing else, I hope she knows this love is forever. Sew, Seamstress, sew and when your fingers ache, and your sewing is done, it's alright to rest because you've given your best.

Many have benefited from your love and the gift you pass on, and there's no doubt it will make us all strong. As your mending comes to an end, don't worry because we'll see you again, on that glorious day when we're reunited with our sweet and dear friend,
"The Seamstress".

Renzie's Park

Everyone has that special place they can go to when confusion sets in and times are hard. Some call it a closet; I call it Renzie's Park.

Such a magnificent place, a place where education is given and meditation is required. It's also a mood changer that picks me up when I'm down and helps me stand when I fall.

It comforts me when I can't get in touch with my father or when he doesn't need to be bothered with something that I can fix.
When I stubble it balances me with thoughts of how things could be, if I just hang in there when my life is at a stall.

It's a place for all seasons, snow covered mountains in the winter, a sweet smelling aroma in the spring; blistering sun rays in the summer and gorgeous colors in the fall, and I have the privilege of calling it my all.

I'm selfish when it comes to sharing its magic, so I ask for forgiveness as I try to keep it for myself. A transformation occurs with every visit I make, all for the good of becoming a better person.

Renzie's Park allows me to bloom with the flowers, sing with the birds and laugh with the clouds as they display images only a child can imagine. It's a place I call my home away from home.

When that time comes and I have to part, I'm never discouraged because I'll take a piece of it with me, tucked away in my heart.

Saying good-bye is never easy, so I'll see you later!

About the Author

Lorenza "Renzie" Thompson, a small town, big idea person, with dreams of one day walking hand in hand with my heavenly father. The creator of situation writing, a form of writing that taps deep into one's heart and soul. When I say I'm blessed, it's not just a figure of speech or a comeback when I'm asked the greeting of the day. It's without a doubt, what's happening right now in my life.

I cherish the little things in life, things like the smell of honeysuckles in the spring air, the wind blowing through the trees. I believe GOD's reason for putting a pen in my hand, is so I can tell not only my journey, but, the stories of those who remain silent, for one reason or another, those who need help, but don't know how or won't ask for it.

As I attempt to, relax, energizes, sooth and massage those who read, live and feel my writing, I hope I help you get through, over and away from whatever bad situation you may be going through, or simply bring more happiness to an already happy life. Just know, you're not alone and help has arrived, just when you thought you couldn't go any further.

GOD has allowed me to endure what some will call pain and agony. I simply see it as growing into what I've been sent here to become, nothing more, nothing less. I'm delighted he has chosen me to help others with my writing, one of many gifts he has given me.

You see, we often forget about the little things in life and become materialistic, but not this person, and if I try to, Heavenly Father, put me in my place. But for now, please allow me to continue and finish this race.

About The Book

Peace Therapy is the beginning of your healing, its therapy for the mind and soul. So, if you're tired of hurting, being depressed, confused or just want the joy and happiness in your life to be magnified, then *Peace Therapy* is just what the doctor ordered.

You will ask yourself, how can anything good come out of my situation? That question will be answered; you may or may not like the outcome, but don't give up. You can't allow "the pause" in your life to have its way.

Peace Therapy will bring up old memories, happy and bad times, love ones and enemies you might have or had. It will show you the mistakes you've made and how to correct them. In order to move on, you must be willing to face and fight whatever brought you to this point.

Help is here, and by working together, I'm sure we can remove the roadblocks and lose the weights we don't have to carry around anymore. Rehabilitation is just another word for pain. One thing for certain, you have to go through it before you can move on. Who ever heard of rehabilitation being fun and painless?

Healing won't be pain free, but it will quench your thirst for knowledge, if that's what you're looking for, it will attempt to answer questions and solve disagreements. Certain areas will take your breathe away, make you cry and laugh, but that's part of healing.

It will massage your pain away, sooth your heart, get rid of all those unwanted thoughts, and magnify your happiness. It's out with the old, in with the new.

So sit back and let *Peace Therapy* guide you through the next phase of your life, good or bad, I'll be with you all the way.
Your session begins now!

www.ingramcontent.com/pod-product-compliance
Lightning Source LLC
Chambersburg PA
CBHW020918290526
45784CB00002BA/604